OXFORD NEUROLOGY LIBRARY

Parkinson's Disease

Edited by

Professor Anthony H.V. Schapira

Head of Department of Clinical Neurosciences,
UCL Institute of Neurology,
National Hospital for Neurology
and Neurosurgery and Royal Free Hospital,
London, UK

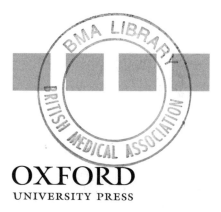

OXFORD
UNIVERSITY PRESS

OXFORD
UNIVERSITY PRESS

Great Clarendon Street, Oxford OX2 6DP

Oxford University Press is a department of the University of Oxford.
It furthers the University's objective of excellence in research, scholarship,
and education by publishing worldwide in

Oxford New York

Auckland Cape Town Dar es Salaam Hong Kong Karachi
Kuala Lumpur Madrid Melbourne Mexico City Nairobi
New Delhi Shanghai Taipei Toronto

With offices in

Argentina Austria Brazil Chile Czech Republic France Greece
Guatemala Hungary Italy Japan Poland Portugal Singapore
South Korea Switzerland Thailand Turkey Ukraine Vietnam

Oxford is a registered trade mark of Oxford University Press
in the UK and in certain other countries

Published in the United States
by Oxford University Press Inc., New York

British Library Cataloguing in Publication Data
Data available

Library of Congress Cataloging in Publication Data
Data available

Typeset by Newgen Imaging Systems (P) Ltd, Chennai, India
Printed in Great Britain
on acid-free paper through
Ashford Colour Press Ltd., Gosport, Hampshire.

ISBN 978–0–19–955063–0

10 9 8 7 6 5 4 3 2

Dedication

This book is dedicated to my wife Laura and daughter Sarah. Their continuing love and support makes all projects such as this possible.

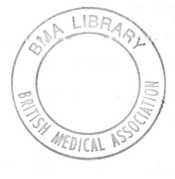

Contents

Preface

Parkinson's disease is the second most common neurodegenerative disease after Alzheimer's disease and its prevalence is rising as the world's population ages. Thus it is inevitable that all physicians will at some point be called upon to diagnose and manage patients with this disorder. This book serves to provide a brief and accessible review of the most important areas of Parkinson's disease from aetiology and diagnosis through to treatment of its various stages. Research in these areas is progressing rapidly and this book seeks to provide an up-to-date review of the most recent advances in the relevant fields. The book is intended for a wide audience that includes the neurologist or geriatrician in training as well as the established physician whose practice may be general or whose specialist interest lies outside of neurology or movement disorders. Particular thanks go to an impressive array of international authors who worked hard to provide excellent and valuable reviews of their respective topics.

Anthony H.V. Schapira

Abbreviations

AAN	American Academy of Neurology
AD	Alzheimer's disease
AuD	autosomal dominant mode
CBGD	corticobasal ganglion degeneration
CDS	continuous dopaminergic stimulation
COMT	catechol-*O*-methyltransferase
CSF	cerebrospinal fluid
CT	computerized tomography
DAT	dopamine transporter
DBS	deep brain stimulation
DLB	dementia with Lewy bodies
DRB	dopamine related behaviours
DRPLA	dentatorubral-pallidoluysian atrophy
ECT	electroconvulsive therapy
ET	essential tremor
FDG	flurodeoxyglucose
GABA	glutamate-amino butyric acid
GAD	glutamic acid decarboxylase
GDNF	glial-derived neurotrophic factor
GPi	globus pallidus interna
ICD	impulse control disorders
IPG	implantable pulse generator
LDR	long duration response
LID	levodopa-induced dyskinesias
MAO	monoamine oxidase
MCI	mild cognitive impairment
MPTP	1-methyl-4-phenyl-1, 2, 3, 6-tetrahydropyridine
MRI	magnetic resonance imaging
MSA	multiple system atrophy
NMDA	*N*-methyl-D-aspartate
NMS	non-motor symptoms

NPH	normal pressure hydrocephalus
OH	orthostatic hypotension
PD	Parkinson's disease
PDD	Parkinson's disease with dementia
PET	positron emission tomography
PKAN	pantothenate kinase associated neurodegeneration
PSP	progressive supranuclear palsy
QoSL-Q	Quality of Sexual Life Questionnaire
RBD	REM sleep behaviour disorder
REM	rapid eye movement
RLS	restless leg syndrome
SCA	spinocerebellar ataxias
SPECT	single photon emission CT
SSRI	selective serotonin reuptake inhibitors
STN	subthalamic nucleus
TCA	tricyclic antidepressants
UPDRS	Unified Parkinson's Disease Rating Scale

Contributors

Charles H. Adler MD PhD
Professor of Neurology, Chair,
Mayo Division of Movement
Disorders,
Mayo Clinic Arizona,
Scottsdale, AZ, USA

Bryan T. Klaasen MD PhD
Movement Disorders Fellow,
Mayo Clinic Arizona,
Scottsdale, AZ, USA

Nico L. Leenders MD PhD
Professor of Neurology,
Department of Neurology,
University Medical Centre Gro-
ningen (UMCG),
Groningen, The Netherlands

Patricia Limousin MD PhD
Reader in Clinical Neurology,
Honorary Consultant,
Institute of Neurology,
National Hospital for Neurology
and Neurosurgery,
London, UK

Irene Martinez-Torres MD
Clinical Research Fellow,
Unit of Functional
Neurosurgery,
Sobell Department,
Institute of Neurology,
London, UK

Shyamal H. Meta MD
Fellow, Movement Disorders
Program,
Department of Neurology,
Medical College of Georgia,
Augusta, GA, USA

Olivier Rascol MD
Clinical Investigation Center and
Departments of Clinical Phar-
macology and Neurosciences,
Faculté de Medicine,
Toulouse, France

Heinz Reichmann MD PhD
Professor and Chair Department
of Neurology,
Dean of Medical Faculty,
University of Dresden,
Dresden, Germany

**Anthony H.V. Schapira
MD DSc**
Head of Department of Clinical
Neurosciences,
UCL Institute of Neurology,
National Hospital for Neurology
and Neurosurgery and Royal
Free Hospital,
London, UK

Anette Schrag MD PhD
Department of Clinical
Neurosciences,
Royal Free Hospital,
University College London,
London, UK

Kapil D. Sethi MD
Professor of Neurology,
Director, Movement Disorders
Program,
Medical College of Georgia,
Augusta, GA, USA

Andrew Siderowf MD
Parkinson's Disease and
Movement Disorder Center,
Philadelphia, PA
and Department of Neurology,
University of Pennsylvania
School of Medicine,
Philadelphia, PA, USA

Matthew B. Stern MD
Penn Neurologic Institute,
Philadelphia, PA, USA

Eng K. Tan MD PhD
Department of Neurology,
Singapore General Hospital,
Singapore

**Jayne R. Wilkinson MD
PhD**
Associate Clinical Director,
Parkinson's Disease and
Movement Disorder Center,
Philadelphia, PA, USA

Chapter 1

Introduction

Anthony H.V. Schapira

The 200-year anniversary of James Parkinson's description of the neurological disorder that was later to bear his name is nearly upon us. It is interesting to reflect on the enormous advances that have been made in our understanding of the clinical features, aetiology, pathology and pathogenesis of this disease, and on the treatments that have become available for sufferers of Parkinson's disease (PD).

Although suspected for many years, recent discoveries have confirmed that there are many causes of PD—at least in terms of genetics. Prior to the identification of the first gene for familial PD our understanding of the cause of PD was based upon epidemiological studies and biochemical analyses of post mortem brain samples. The former suggested that certain chemicals, e.g. pesticides, herbicides, 1-methyl 4-phenyl 1, 2, 3, 6 tetrahydropyridine and some occupations e.g. farmers, teachers, increased the risk for PD, although these findings were not reproduced in all studies. Biochemical studies identified mitochondrial dysfunction and oxidative stress as important components of pathogenesis; inflammation and protein handling were also recognized as contributing to neuronal loss. The discovery of alpha-synuclein mutations and multiplications as a cause of PD and that this protein was an important component of Lewy bodies focussed attention on protein aggregation as a contributor to PD. Subsequent findings again highlighted mitochondrial abnormalities as central to PD causation including the description of the mitochondrial proteins PINK1 and DJ1 as PD-causing genes, and that parkin, another cause of familial PD, had important mitochondrial interactions. The most common cause of PD identified to date is mutations of the LRRK2 gene. The G2019S mutation alone accounts for up to 40% of PD in North African Berber Arabs and up to 5% of apparently sporadic PD in some other communities. Other genes will no doubt be discovered and it is very likely that association or 'risk' genes will become recognized as important factors in PD causation. For instance, glucocerebrosidase mutations appear to be a significant risk factor for PD.

Genetics clearly plays an important role in PD aetiology. Although the environment may serve to modify penetrance and expression of these genes, major associations between environmental factors and PD await identification.

The clinical phenotype of PD continues to be of major interest and recent attention has focussed particularly on the PD prodrome, i.e. the development of symptoms and signs prior to diagnosis. It has become clear that a proportion of patients may experience a combination or permutation of olfactory loss, rapid eye movement sleep behaviour disorder, depression, constipation, and possibly impaired colour vision discrimination. It is hoped that these clinical features, perhaps combined with biochemical or easily accessible imaging markers, might constitute 'biomarkers' that could allow identification of at risk individuals who would be suitable for early treatment with neuroprotective drugs.

The diagnosis of PD remains a clinical one—based on the motor features of the disease. Imaging, of the dopamine transporter for instance, may be useful to distinguish PD from essential tremor or dystonic tremor, but does not reliably separate the parkinsonian syndromes, e.g. multiple system atrophy or progressive supranuclear palsy from each other or from PD.

Study of the clinical progression of PD has also highlighted the non-motor symptoms as a major determinant of the quality of life of patients, as well as the need for institutional placement and life expectancy. Cognitive disturbances including dementia, confusion and hallucinations, depression and a range of autonomic abnormalities can develop early in PD, but typically manifest later in disease progression. Treatment for these problems remains limited and unsatisfactory.

The treatment of PD remains focussed on the motor symptoms and comprises mainly dopaminergic therapy. Levodopa is still the mainstay of treatment and can be combined with both dopa-decarboxylase and catechol-O-methyl transferase inhibitors to increase its half life and effectiveness. Dopamine agonists continue to evolve with new compounds and new preparations including skin patches and once-a-day oral formulations are now available. Monoamine oxidase inhibition is a useful strategy for symptom relief in both early and late disease. Infusions of apomorphine or levodopa are helpful for advanced PD. Non-medical therapies in the form of deep brain stimulation or ablative procedures (now used less commonly) remain an important option in late disease.

The timing of treatment initiation for PD has been a topic of interest and debate. Although traditionally treatment was withheld until the patient suffered sufficient disability, the availability of modern drugs and an increasing recognition that earlier treatment may confer long term benefit have shifted initiation to earlier in the disease course.

Neuroprotection remains an important goal for PD research. Advances in our understanding of the aetiopathogensis of PD have provided a multitude of compounds that may have potential in slowing the progression of PD. The challenge is how to test these in patients and demonstrate a modification of the progression of the disease. In the absence of a recognized biomarker of disease progression other than clinical (motor) dysfunction, clinical trial design has turned to delayed start comparisons to demonstrate an effect with symptomatic agents. Trials of rasagiline have shown that this drug can provide a better motor outcome when given earlier rather than later. The mechanism of this effect remains open to debate.

Based upon an impressive series of advances over the last 50 years, it seems reasonable for PD patients and their families to be optimistic about new discoveries relating to the cause and prevention.

Chapter 2

Causes of Parkinson's disease: genetics, environment and pathogenesis

Eng K. Tan and Heinz Reichmann

Key points

- Parkinson's Disease (PD) is a neurodegenerative disorder of complex aetiology where both genetic and environmental factors play a role in its pathophysiology
- A number of disease-causing genes have been identified in both familial and sporadic forms of PD, and some environmental factors have been shown to modulate the risk of the disease
- Regardless of its underlying etiology, both in vitro and animal studies have suggested abnormalities in mitochondrial function, oxidative and nitrosative stress, accumulation of aberrant or misfolded proteins, and ubiquitin-proteasome system dysfunction represent the principal molecular pathways that underpin its pathophysiology.

2.1 Introduction

The term 'Idiopathic Parkinson's Disease' (PD) applies to PD patients without an overt cause of the disease and differentiates them from those who have a Parkinson syndrome as a consequence of trauma, stroke, intoxication, medication, and inflammation (encephalitis), to name just a few. The term idiopathic is a noble one for a situation where no definite reason for the occurrence of Parkinsonism can be found. Nonetheless, there is an increasing number of patients who develop Parkinsonian symptoms due to genetic abnormalities and in future they may have to be excluded from the group of idiopathic

PD. Nevertheless, we will describe the latest genetic findings in detail. On the other hand, there is a strong possibility that PD may be due to environmental factors (viruses, bacteria, toxins) if we take the findings of Braak and coworkers seriously. They stress that the earliest typical PD abnormalities (such as Lewy bodies, Lewy neuritis, α-synuclein) occur in the Meissner and Auerbach plexus and in the olfactory bulb (Braak et al., 2006). This explains the clinical observation that constipation and hyposmia are early symptoms of PD (Müller et al., 2002) and that gastric ulcers are often followed 10–20 years later by PD (*Helicobacter jejuni* infection). In addition, we know that cell death of dopaminergic neurons is associated with a cascade of cellular events such as energy crisis, oxidative stress, glial inflammation, proteasomal abnormalities, and protein aggregation (Figure 2.1).

It is a major problem that at present we do not know which of these factors are the primary ones; therefore any neuroprotective therapy is difficult to plan.

2.2 Genetic causes

2.2.1 Discovery of causative genes

The age-old debate regarding the relative contribution of gene-environment interaction in PD has generated considerable interest within the scientific community. The unravelling of the human genome project brings optimism that an unequivocal answer will be clarified soon. In 1983, the discovery of MPTP (methyl-4-phenyl-1, 2, 3, 6-tetrahydropyridine)-induced Parkinsonism in intravenous drug users led

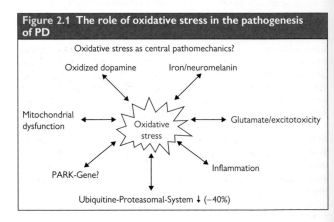

Figure 2.1 **The role of oxidative stress in the pathogenesis of PD**

Oxidative stress as central pathomechanics?

Oxidized dopamine

Iron/neuromelanin

Mitochondrial dysfunction

Oxidative stress

Glutamate/excitotoxicity

PARK-Gene?

Inflammation

Ubiquitine-Proteasomal-System ↓ (−40%)

many to speculate that environmental factors could be the primary etiology of PD. However, in 1997 a missense mutation in the α-synuclein gene was found to be associated with the disease in some families with autosomal dominant (AuD) mode of inheritance of parkinsonism. Since then, investigators have managed to identify at least 13 genetic loci and seven disease-causing genes have been uncovered.

2.2.2 Nomenclature

The naming of pathogenic or susceptibility genes follows a nomenclature with numerical assignment starting with PARK1, the first reported gene (α-synuclein). The pathogenic genes are either associated with autosomal recessive (PARK2; PARKIN, PARK6; PINK1, PARK7; DJ-1), or autosomal dominant mode of inheritance (PARK1; alpha synuclein, PARK8; LRRK2, PARK9; ATP13A2). More recently, mutations of the GIGYF2 gene at the PARK11 locus have been reported (Table 2.1).

2.2.3 Prevalence of genetic mutations

The prevalence of PARK1, PARK7 and PARK9 mutations is low (<1%) in most populations.

Importantly, Parkin (PARK2) accounts for up to 50% and 15–20% of autosomal recessive and young onset sporadic PD. Mutations in the leucine-rich repeat kinase 2 (*LRRK2, PARK8*) are the most frequent known cause of familial autosomal dominant PD. The common G2019S mutation accounts for 3-7% of familial PD and 1–3% in sporadic PD in several ethnic populations, with highest prevalence (up to 40%) in North Africans and Ashkanezi Jews. However, some of these figures have to be interpreted with caution as they may not genuinely reflect prevalence in the general population but rather those in specialist clinics and tertiary referral centers.

2.2.3.1 *Differentiating 'familial Parkinsonism' from 'idiopathic' PD*

Mutation carriers of PARK1, and PARK9 generally have atypical features (such as very early onset of disease (<20 years) and presence of other movement disorders) that are not found in most of the 'idiopathic' forms of PD. More recent studies have suggested that carriers of PARK6 and PARK7 have clinically features similar to young onset (<45 years) PD, such as excellent response to dopaminergic agent and early dopamine related drug complications,

Clinically, one cannot differentiate between carriers and non-carriers of the common recurrent LRRK2 mutation (G2019S) and the surprisingly high frequency of mutations in sporadic cases questions the view that the genetic forms are different from the common garden variety and should be termed separately as 'familial parkinsonism' as distinct from 'idiopathic' PD.

Table 2.1 Pathogenic genes in Parkinson's disease

Locus/ Mode of inheritance	Gene	Mutations	Possible risk variants	Protein function
PARK1 & PARK4 (4q21) (AuD)	SNCA	Dominant A30P, E46K and A53T; genomic duplication/triplication	Promoter polymorphism (rep1) increases risk	Dopamine transmission and synaptic vesicle dynamics
PARK2 (6q25.2-27) (AR)	Parkin	Numerous recessive homozygote/compound heterozygote missense, truncating, exon deletion/duplication/ triplication	Promoter polymorphism may increase risk	Ubiquitin E3 ligase
PARK5 (4p14) (AuD)	UCHL1	Heterozygous I93M	S18Y variant may protect in younger subjects	Ubiquitin hydrolase
PARK6 (1p35-36) (AR)	PINK1	Various recessive missense, exon deletion	–	Mitochondria kinase
PARK7 (1p36) (AR)	DJ1	Various recessive homozygous/compound heterozygous missense, exon deletion	–	Oxidative stress response
PARK8 (12p12) (AuD)	LRRK2	Numerous dominant missense	G2385R and R1628P increase risk among Asians	Protein kinase
PARK11 (2p21.2) (AuD)	GIGYF2	Numerous dominant missense	–	Insulin signaling

2.2.3.2 Genetic risk factors

For pathogenic genes, one can invariably demonstrate the co-segregation of the genotype and phenotype in family and case control studies, and the presence of a disruption of biological function of the protein as a result of the mutation. However, demonstration of genetic risk/ protective variants (polymorphic variants) can be problematic. A polymorphism refers to a variation in the DNA that is too common to be due merely to new mutation. A polymorphism must have a frequency of at least 1% in the general population. The link between a polymorphic variant and a specific disease trait is usually carried out in a genetic association study where the frequency of the variant among diseased group is compared to a group of unrelated healthy controls. However, genetic association studies are confounded by various methodological problems. Genetic association studies in PD have frequently given conflicting findings, likely because of inadequate sample size, bias in selecting only individual polymorphic loci of susceptibility genes so that background genetic variations are not systematically studied and population stratification. Some of these problems can be surmounted by using sib-pairs, genetic isolates, whole genome amplication and multi-center meta-analysis of pooled data. Despite these limitations, some genetic variants have been identified to modulate the risk of PD. Notably, the common variants of LRRK2 (G2385R, R1628P) have been consistently shown to increase the risk of PD by two-fold in various populations among Asians. While the exact pathophysiologic role of these risk variants is currently unknown, the identification of these variants may one day facilitate the development of clinical, bioimaging, genetic or other biological biomarkers, potentially useful in the monitoring and neuroprotective therapy in asymptomatic carriers.

2.2.3.3 *Genetic testing in PD*

Genetic testing in the broadest sense refers to laboratory studies of blood (DNA) or other tissues for the purpose of identifying disorders that have an underlying genetic abnormality.

Genetic testing allows early confirmation of diagnosis and genetic counselling. It can be helpful for selecting specific patients for clinical drug trials and can provide a better understanding of the pathogenesis and long-term clinical outcome of the disease.

So is there a role for genetic testing in PD? Unfortunately there are a number of concerns at present to unequivocally recommend this as a routine clinical service. One of the cardinal problems is there is not enough scientific data for us to properly advise and counsel our patients or their relatives on the progression and prognosis of the disease. The pathogenicity of a number of mutations has not been clarified, and carriers may never develop, or have a low risk of developing the disease in their lifetime. Some investigators have suggested that genetic testing may have a role in patients who have a family history of PD, or in those with very young age of onset where a family member has already been diagnosed to carry a known mutation. In such scenarios, the patients may request for genetic confirmation for social and medical reasons. As genetic testing may have serious implications, it should be performed only after careful consideration and a genetic counseling process involving doctors, professional counsellors, and the affected patient and family.

2.3 **Environmental causes of Parkinson's disease**

There is a considerable list of drugs and toxins inducing Parkinsonism. The most important ones are neuroleptics, antiemetics, reserpine, manganese and carbon monoxide. The intake of *Annona muricata* caused a Parkinson syndrome on Guadeloupe. Methyl-phenyl-tetrahydro-pyridinium is the most important toxin which inhibits complex I of the respiratory chain in dopaminergic neurons of the substantia nigra and which leads to PD in humans. Therefore MPTP is the most important tool to create an animal model of PD. This is based upon its selective affinity for dopaminergic neurons in the substantia nigra. The inhibition of complex I leads to an increase of reactive oxygen species and a decrease of ATP production. Similar results can be obtained with the application of another complex I inhibitor, rotenone. Our own group (Bringmann et al., 1995) identified the toxin TaClo (which may be generated from chloralhydrate, used as a sleeping pill, and trichloroethylene, used as an organic solvent, for example in dry cleaners). Since both these toxins and medication such as neuroleptics, flunarizine, cimetidine, and others are not the cause of the disease in the majority of PD patients, there may be other environmental factors which may even be present at pregnancy. In rural areas of the US, where farmers use large amounts of herbicides and pesticides and drink water from their own wells, a higher prevalence of PD has been reported (Brown et al. 2005, Brighina et al. 2008). Apart from these findings, there are no other conclusive reports about possible environmental toxins causing PD. Recently, bacteria have also been discussed as potential agents, because their endotoxins, lipopolysaccharides, may also be also harmful to the substantia nigra. In particular, bacterial vaginoses with *Gardnerella vaginalis* are suspected to induce an abnormal development of the nigrostriatal system in the fetal period. In this context, the hypothesis that *Helicobacter jejuni* may lead to the development of PD should be reemphasized. It is speculated that these bacteria may activate glial cells and produce proinflammatory cytokines thus reducing neurotrophic factors.

2.4 **Pathogenesis of dopaminergic cell death**

2.4.1 **Energy crisis**

There is an increasing body of evidence that PD patients present with a complex I defect in the substantia nigra (Schapira et al., 1989; Janetzky et al., 1994). Unlike other disorders of the mitochondrial respiratory chain this defect only presents with a reduction of complex I activity to 60–70% of controls. It could be shown that in synaptosomes even a decrease in complex I activity of more than 25% leads to a considerable reduction of ATP-production. Over many years the damage caused by mitochondrial dysfunction accumulates and causes not only a reduction of ATP production but also impairs membrane potential and energy metabolism, leading to increased free radical production. Since the subunits of complex I are encoded both by the mitochondrial and the nuclear genome, it was interesting to test where the complex I deficiency arises from. So far, no specific point mutation or common deletion have been found neither in the mt nor in the ncDNA. Nevertheless, there is stronger evidence for alterations of mtDNA than of ncDNA (rho-zero cell analyses). In addition to a complex I defect, some patients also present with a minor complex III deficiency which may further worsen the aforementioned malfunctions. As a result of increased free radical formation the mitochondrial DNA and to a lesser extent the nuclear DNA are impaired by hydroxyl radicals. This leads to mutations of the mitochondrial DNA which will be described in detail in the next paragraph.

2.4.2 **Radical formation, oxidative stress**

Free radicals such as the hydroxyl radical are not only generated with complex I and III deficiencies but also with reduced levels of glutathione and glutathione peroxidase activity, and increased iron concentrations in the dopaminergic neurons. Via the so-called Fenton reaction this leads to increased concentrations of hydroxyl radicals. These radicals not only damage DNA molecules by forming 8-OH-deoxyguanosine, but they also induce lipid peroxidation and open up double bonds which allows Ca-ions to penetrate the cell walls and activate Ca-dependent nucleases and proteases. DNA abnormalities then further impair the synthesis of the respiratory chain complexes and add to the energy crisis. In this context, it could be shown that mitochondrial DNA is deleted or shows point mutations in a considerable number of dopaminergic neurons (Bender et al. 2006). Since the mitochondrial genome encodes for 13 subunits of the respiratory chain and is located in close proximity to the site of free radical production in the mitochondria, it is particularly prone to oxidative damage. Another source of free radical production is activated microglia as discussed below. Considering the various genetic defects leading to PD it is particularly interesting that three of the recessive PD genes are linked to mitochondrial function. Parkin (PARK2) is the most frequently mutated gene in patients with early-onset PD. In Parkin mutants muscle degeneration and mitochondrial pathology could be demonstrated. PINK-1 localizes to the mitochondria and DJ-1 is a sensor for oxidative stress and also linked to mitochondria. These findings also support the assumptions shown in Figure 2.1.

2.4.3 **Protein aggregation**

All neurodegenerative disorders are characterized by the aggregation of misfolded proteins. In Alzheimer's disease, it is β-amyloid and in PD it is α-synuclein. The function of α-synuclein is still not fully understood, but it seems to play an important role in the maintenance of cell membrane integrity. The degradation of defective, oxidized or no longer necessary proteins is normally accomplished by the ubiquitine-proteasomal system. Ubiquitination and degradation of α-synuclein, however, do not utilize the proteasomal system (compare with Section 2.4.2), which leads to the accumulation of α-synuclein in Lewy bodies and causes problems with cell trafficking. Not only genetic defects of α-synuclein, however, may cause PD but also patients overexpressing α-synuclein (three copies instead of two) develop PD in their fifties whilst those with four copies develop PD in their thirties (Singleton, 2003). This suggests early breakdown of the proteasomal system. McNaught and colleagues (2006) claim that dysfunction of the proteasomal system is one of the major reasons for dopaminergic cell death. Impairment of the proteasomal system causes accumulation of oxidized proteins which may give rise to the formation of Lewy bodies, to free radical production, to the induction of the caspase cascade and eventually apoptosis. Recent findings indicate a 40% reduction in proteasomal activity in the substantia nigra from PD patients.

2.4.4 **Inflammation, glial reactions in PD**

It is known that microglia constitutes about 10% of all glial cells. The highest concentration of microglia is found in the substantia nigra. Microglia seems to act as a cell patrol and microglial cells are able to respond to any cellular injury very rapidly. Immunohistochemistry shows activated microglia in post mortem brains from most PD patients. According to McGeer and McGeer (2008), PD is not an autoimmune disease but, because of the activated microglia, is rather an autotoxic disorder. In this context, it is interesting that in regular NSAID users the development of PD is reduced by 55%. Alpha-synuclein can induce glial reactions. It is quite possible that leaky dopaminergic neurons (oxidative stress, necrosis and apoptosis of dopaminergic neurons) will enhance the delivery and presentation of α-synuclein to microglia which will induce inflammation. The PET marker [11C]-(R)-PK11195 can be employed to demonstrate activated microglia in humans. Using this method Ouchi et al. (2005) found an increase of activated microglia and a decreased activity of dopamine transporters in PD patients. Activated microglia produces large amounts of superoxide radicals which add to the hydroxyl radicals produced in the Fenton reaction. The upregulation of microglial receptors (such as the laminin-receptor) observed in PD may represent a new target for the treatment of PD. In addition, there are reports that microglia may express D_1 and D_2 dopaminergic receptors and that dopamine agonists may prevent microglia from producing pro-inflammatory cytokines.

The discussion of cerebral inflammation would be incomplete without including the role of astrocytes. Far from being completely sedentary, they move towards cellular injuries and segregate them off. It has been shown that astrocytes in the substantia nigra express ICAM-1 which will attract activated microglia. Together with abnormal α-synuclein, this will enhance inflammatory responses. Conversely, astrocytes can produce glial-cell derived neurotrophic factor (GDNF) and mesencephalic astrocyte-derived neurotrophic factor (MANF) which are both neurotrophic factors for dopaminergic neurons. Finally, actrocytes also express DJ-1 which is impaired in PARK7. In this context, it is of interest that microglia, astrocytes and oligodendroglia can express leucine-rich repeat kinase 2 (LRRK2) specific mRNA. Mutations of LRRK2 have been discussed in great detail in the section on genetics (compare Section 2.2).

In conclusion, there is convincing data on the role of microglia and astrocytes in PD and it is therefore tempting to speculate whether early and continuous use of NSAID may prevent or modify the disease. Furthermore, substances like valproic acid which can induce the synthesis of neurotrophic factors, or dopamine agonists which may attenuate inflammatory processes, might also be beneficial for patients.

2.4.5 Aging

There is no doubt that ageing is the most important risk factor for the development of PD. Besides many other factors, ageing produces disturbances of iron homeostasis, leads to a decrease of energy production and an increase of reactive oxygen species concentrations, causes alterations of the cytoskeleton and induces chromatin changes. All these parameters are important for the development of PD. Thus, the longer our life expectancy the more prone we will be to develop PD.

2.4.6 Dopamine toxicity

Dopamine has a high potential to oxidize other substrates and requires adequate regulation of production and degradation. As a consequence of decreased concentrations of reduced glutathione and glutathione peroxidase, dopamine may be transformed to hydrogen peroxide which in turn will produce hydroxyl radicals via the Fenton reaction because of the increased iron concentrations. In cell culture dopamine can induce apoptosis. The most important factor responsible for this seems to be the generation of reactive oxygen species induced by dopamine. Under normal conditions dopamine is therefore sequestered into vesicles prior to its release into the synaptic cleft and subsequent stimulation of the dopamine receptors.

Whilst the debate is still open if dopamine itself is involved in the death of dopaminergic neurons, it has to be considered that glial cells have a high capacity to scavenge free radicals. Currently, most researchers believe that at least in the early stages of the disease dopamine does not play a major role in cell death.

2.4.7 **Iron and neuromelanin**

Riederer and others have shown that total iron content is significantly increased in the substantia nigra of PD patients (Riederer *et al.*, 1989). Under normal conditions, basal ganglia contain substantial amounts of iron, and an increase in iron III catalyses the Fenton reaction towards the formation of hydroxyl radicals. It is therefore convincing that iron is a major player in oxidative stress. Iron is bound to ferritin which is found in activated microglia, for instance. In dopaminergic cells this function is taken over by neuromelanin which also binds iron. It is speculated that in PD the binding capacity of neuromelanin for iron is too low which causes iron to be cleaved and leads to oxidative stress. In this context, it is interesting that in the substantia nigra the cells best preserved from degeneration are the melanin-containing cells.

2.4.8 **Glutamate and excitotoxicity**

Glutamate is an important neurotransmitter for the control of movement and also acts at the small spiny neurons of the striatum. In addition, substantia nigra pars compacta also contains glutamatergic receptors to receive stimulatory input from the cortex and subthalamic nucleus. Because of the characteristic disinhibition of the subthalamic nucleus in PD glutamatergic overstimulation may cause excitotoxic stress (Rodriguez *et al.*, 1998). Eventually glutamate causes depolarisation, Ca-influx and cell death. In addition, glutamate can induce oxidative stress via the NO.-radical. Another site of action is the NMDA receptor. Due to the complex I defect the Mg^{2+} blockade of the NMDA receptor is no longer possible which leads to a continuous influx of Ca^{2+}-ions that is further increased by glutamate release. These findings, however, still require definite neuropathological proof.

References and further reading

Bender A., Krishnan K.J., Morris C.M., Taylor D.A., Reeve A.K., Perry, R.H., Jaros E., Hersheson J.S., Betts J., Klopstock T., Taylor R.W., Turnbull D.M. (2006) High levels of mitochondrial DNA deletions in substantia nigra neurons in aging and Parkinson disease. *Nat. Genet.* **38**, 515–17.

Braak H. DeVos R.A.I., Bohl J., Del Tredici K. (2006) Gastric α-synuclein immunoreactive inclusions in Meissner's and Auerbach's plexuses in cases staged for Parkinson's disease-related brain pathology. *Neurosci. Lett.* **396**, 67–72.

Brighina L., Frigerio R., Schneider N.K. (2008) α-synuclein, pesticides, and Parkinson disease: a case-control study. *Neurology*. **70**, 1461–9.

Bringmann, G., God, R., Feineis D., Wesemann W., Riederer P., Rausch W.-D., Reichmann H., Sontag K.-H. (1995). The TaClo concept: 1-trichloromethyl-1,2,3,4-tetahydro--carboline (TaClo), a new toxin for dopaminergic neurons. *J. Neural Transm.* [Suppl] **46**, 235–244

Brown R.C., Lockwood, A.H., and Sonawane B.R. (2005) Neurodegenerative diseases: an overview of environmental risk factors. *Environ. Health Perspect.* **113**, 1250–6.

Janetzky B., Hauck S., Youdim M.B., Riederer P., Jellinger K., Pantucek F., Zöchling R., Boissl K.W., Reichmann H. (1994) Unaltered aconitase activity, but decreased complex I activity in substantia nigra pars compacta of patients with Parkinson's disease. *Neurosci Lett* **169**, 126–8.

McNaught K.S., Jackson T., Jnobaptiste R., Kapustin A., Olanow C.W. (2006) Proteasomal dysfunction in sporadic Parkinson's disease. *Neurology*, **66**, S37–S49.

McGeer P.L. and McGeer E.G. (2008). Glial reactions in Parkinson's disease. *Movement Disord.* **23**, 474–83.

Müller A., Reichmann H., Livermore A., Hummel T. (2002) Olfactory function in idiopathic Parkinson's disease (IPD): results from cross-sectional studies in IPD patients and long-term follow-up of de novo IPD patients. *J. Neural Transm.* **109**, 805– 11.

Ouichi Y., Yoshikawa E., Sekine Y. (2005) Microglial activation and dopamine terminal loss in early Parkinson's disease. *Ann. Neurol.* **57**, 168-175.

Riederer P., Sofic E., Rausch W.D., Schmidt D., Reynolds G.P. *et al.* (1989) Transition metals, ferritin, glutathione, and ascorbic acid in parkinsonian brains. *J. Neurochem.* **52**, 515–20.

Rodriguez M.C., Obeso J.A., and Olanow W.C. (1998) Subthalamic nucleus-mediated excitotoxicity in Parkinson's disease: a target for neuroprotection. *Ann. Neurol.* **44**, S175–S188.

Schapira A.H., Cooper J.M., Dexter D., Clark J.B., Jenner P., Marsden C.D. (1989) Mitochondrial complex I deficiency in Parkinson's disease. *Lancet* I, 1269.

Singleton A.B., Farrer M., Johnston J., Singleton A., Hague S., Kachergus J., Hulihan M., Peuralinna T., Dutra A., Nussbaum R., Lincoln S., Crawley A., Hanson M., Maraganore D., Adler C., Cookson M.R., Muenter M., Baptista M., Miller C., Balncato J., Hardy J., Gwinn-Hardy K (2003) Alpha-synuclein locus triplication causes Parkinson's disease. *Science* 302, 841.

Tan E.K. (2007) The role of common genetic risk variants in Parkinson disease. *Clin Genet.* **72**(5), 387–93.

Tan E.K., Skipper L.M. (2007) Pathogenic mutations in Parkinson disease. *Hum Mutat.* **28**(7), 641–53.

Chapter 3

Clinical features: motor and nonmotor

Matthew B. Stern and Andrew Siderowf

> **Key points**
> - Parkinson's disease (PD) is characterized by motor features and non-motor features, both of which can cause significant disability
> - The cardinal motor features of PD are bradykinesia, rigidity, resting tremor, and postural instability
> - Motor symptoms of PD begin insidiously and progress gradually throughout the course of the disease
> - The most commonly disabling non-motor features of PD are neuropsychiatric: dementia, depression or drug-induced psychosis
> - Other non-motor features of PD include: autonomic dysfunction, sleep disturbance and sensory complaints.

3.1 Introduction

The cardinal features of Parkinson's disease (PD) include bradykinesia, rigidity, resting tremor, and postural instability. The non-motor aspects of PD include neuropsychiatric disturbances, loss of smell, and autonomic dysfunction, among others. In many cases, the non-motor symptoms are the source of disability, loss of quality of life, and catalyst to placement in nursing homes. Given their non-specificity, their relationship to PD is often only made after motor symptoms/signs have been identified.

3.2 Motor features

The cardinal motor symptoms of PD (bradykinesia, rigidity, resting tremor, and postural instability) develop insidiously and occur with marked individual variability, both in symptom combination, and

Table 3.1 Motor features of Parkinson's disease. This table shows the timing of motor symptoms across the stages of PD

	Early PD	Moderate PD	Advanced PD
Tremor	X	X	X
Rigidity	X	X	X
Bradykinesia	X	X	X
Postural instability			X
Motor fluctuations		X	X

temporal sequence (Table 3.1). Typically, motor symptoms present in an asymmetrical fashion, often in one limb. Subsequently, symptoms spread to the ipsilateral limb, and then to the contralateral limbs and body. Diagnosis of PD is based on clinical phenomenology. The presence of symptoms is termed parkinsonism, and factors such as insidious onset, slowly progressive course, asymmetry, presence of rest tremor, good response to levodopa, and lack of other secondary causes, lead the clinician to arrive at a diagnosis of idiopathic Parkinson's disease.

Bradykinesia. Bradykinesia, or slowness of movement, is considered by many to be the defining feature of PD and is required by many diagnostic criteria. The onset of this symptom is subtle, and may manifest nonspecifically in patients whom report weakness or fatigue. Loss of facial expression, decreased blink rate, and overall loss of spontaneous movement may be noted. Symptoms often develop distally, and a loss of dexterity may be reported. Handwriting may become smaller (micrographia) and inability to pick up the feet can cause shuffling. A delay in initiating movements frequently occurs, known as 'freezing'. A common example of this is freezing of gait. This phenomenon occurs in more advanced disease and represents difficulty initiating gait; or hesitations, particularly in confined spaces (i.e. doorways). The patient's history often provides much evidence for the presence of this symptom. The evaluating clinician can observe these features by simple observation. However, observing sequential movements for slowness, dampened amplitude or an irregular rhythm provides unequivocal evidence of bradykinesia.

Rigidity. Rigidity is a state of hypertonicity with unvarying resistance to passive movement. This smooth, 'lead pipe' resistance is independent of velocity, differentiating this finding from spasticity. Patients with PD have 'cog-wheel' rigidity. Cogwheeling is a common finding on examination, and is thought to be the superimposition of tremor on existing rigidity. Common complaints caused by rigidity are difficulty standing from the seated position and rolling over in bed. Postural and/or limb deformities are also a function of increased muscle tone, and termed dystonia. Rigidity is detected by passive movement of the limbs and head/neck. This symptom is accentuated by asking the patient to use the contralateral limb or engage in mental activation.

Tremor. The hallmark tremor of PD is characterized as a slow 4–6 Hz tremor occurring at rest, dissipating with use of the affected limb(s). Based on its appearance, tremor of the fingers is often described as 'pill-rolling'. In addition to the limbs, tremor can occur in the chin, jaw and tongue. In more advanced stages of the disease a postural and/or action tremor may be evident as well. The resting tremor of PD usually begins intermittently; therefore careful observation should be made to detect its presence. Observing the patient walk, contralateral limb activation and mental activations are all means to illicit subtle intermittent resting tremor.

Postural instability. Postural instability is sometimes included as a fourth cardinal feature. Postural instability results from axial rigidity and bradykinesia as well as loss of the postural or righting reflexes, and typically occurs later in the course of the disease. Postural instability is often accompanied by difficulty with gait including shuffling, difficulty starting and maintaining gait (gait freezing), and festination. Festination is a gait disturbance characterized by short, rapid and accelerating steps and the inability to stop. These postural and gait problems lead to loss of independence, falls and fractures. Historical information will often suffice as evidence of this symptom. Additionally, clinicians can perform a pull test to evaluate the patient's ability to resist retropulsion.

Motor complications. With more advanced disease, patients with PD can develop motor complications. The most common is wearing off, which is defined as loss of the quality of response to dopaminergic medications several hours after the last dose. Patients with advanced PD may experience sudden and unpredictable periods of 'wearing off'. Dyskinesias are also a common and motor complication. These hyperkinetic movements are associated with dopaminergic supplementation and reflect a transient period of dopaminergic excess. Found in moderate and advanced disease, they are also a symptom of the inability to buffer exogenous dopamine. Dyskinesias may be a source of embarrassment, pain and disability.

Progression of motor features. The motor symptoms of PD develop insidiously, and are initially mild (see Table 3.1). It is common for patients to reflect back in time, often months or even years, to symptoms/signs noted prior to diagnosis. Reduced arm swing, shuffled gait, stooped posture, softened voice, decreased facial expressivity or blink rate, small writing and general loss of spontaneous movement are often noted. Progression in PD is universal. The worsening occurs gradually and the rate is highly variable. Mortality is not dramatically increased. Typically there is a period of two to three years when treatment with dopaminergic agents results in excellent control of symptoms. After five years of levodopa treatment, motor complications may develop. After a number of years, the emergence of levodopa-resistant symptoms such as freezing, falling, and dementia, cause significant disability. Older age, rigidity, and hypokinesia as presenting symptoms are predictors of more rapidly progressive disease. Any abrupt onset or change in symptom severity or rate of progression should be regarded as atypical, and further diagnostic consideration is needed.

3.3 Non-motor features of PD

Non-motor aspects of PD are increasingly recognized as a major contributor to overall disability. These non-motor features include neuropsychiatric, autonomic and sensory abnormalities (see Table 3.2). Many non-motor features of PD, particularly dementia, occur later in the disease course.

Neuropsychiatric. There are three major categories of neuropsychiatric problems associated with PD: cognitive impairment, affective disturbance (including anxiety and depression) and psychosis. Impulse control disorders (ICDs) are a distinct, treatment related neuropsychiatric manifestation of PD.

Cognitive impairment is common in PD. A substantial portion of newly diagnosed PD patients will have some evidence of cognitive impairment, and up to 80% of patients will develop dementia over the

Table 3.2 Non-motor features of PD. This table shows major categories of non-motor problems associated with PD

Neuropsychiatric
• Cognitive impairment
• Depression
• Psychosis
• Impulse control disorder
Sleep
• Insomnia
• Daytime sleepiness
• REM sleep behavior disturbance
Autonomic
• Gastro-intestinal
• Genito-urinary
• Circulatory
Sensory
• Pain
• Olfactory dysfunction
• Visual complaints

course of the disease. Compared to patients with Alzheimer's disease (AD), patients with PD have a less profound memory impairment relative to other problems, and more difficulty with planning and mental flexibility ('executive function'). Slowing of mental processing and delayed response-time is common.

There is no definitive treatment of cognitive problems in PD. It is appropriate to discontinue medications that may worsen cognitive function, particularly anti-cholinergics. Cholinesterase inhibitors (rivastigmine) have been shown to improve cognition in patients with PD and dementia. Small-scale trials have suggested a benefit for memantine. However, this has not been confirmed in a large-scale clinical trial.

Unlike cognitive decline, which is a late manifestation of PD, depression may occur at any stage. Approximately 30–50% of PD patients will experience depression at some point during their illness. Social withdrawal and apathy are common co-morbid features associated with depression in PD. Depression in PD may be overlooked because it tends to be hidden by motor slowing and loss of facial expression. As a result, under-diagnosis is a major barrier to appropriate treatment. There is no consensus on the best choice of anti-depressant to use for PD patients. Recent data suggests that tricyclic anti-depressants (nortryptiline) may be at least as effective as selective serotonin reuptake inhibitors (SSRIs).

Anxiety and panic attacks occur as affective manifestations of PD. These anxiety symptoms may occur in isolation or as part of PD-related depression. Treatment of anxiety may include benzodiazepines or SSRIs. Anxiety may also occur as an end-of-dose phenomenon due to falling levels of dopaminergic medications. In this case, anxiety is a psychiatric correlated of 'wearing off' of the motor benefit from dopaminergic medications. A careful history is helpful in identifying this problem, which can be managed in the same way as classic motor fluctuations.

Psychosis is the third major neuropsychiatric problem in PD. Psychosis usually manifests as formed visual hallucinations in the setting of dopaminergic therapy. However, patients with parkinsonism and prominent dementia may have visual hallucinations without dopaminergic treatment. Hallucinations are often well-formed images of children or small animals that are rarely threatening, and cause surprisingly little distress to the patient. Patients with cognitive impairment have increased difficulty in recognizing that the hallucinations are not real, and may attempt to interact with them.

Management of psychosis in PD begins with reduction of offending medications including amantadine, anti-cholinergics and dopamine agonists. Levodopa dose should be lowered after other medications have been removed. If hallucinations persist despite aggressive medication reduction, clozapine or quetiapine may be used. Clozapine treatment requires frequent blood monitoring due to risk of agranulocytopenia. 'Typical' anti-psychotic medications such as haloperidol, risperidone and olanzapine should not be used in PD patients.

Impulse control disorders (ICDs) are an additional neuropsychiatric manifestation of PD. ICDs in PD include pathological gambling, shopping, excessive eating and hypersexuality. The major risk factor for ICDs is treatment with dopaminergic medication, particularly dopamine agonists (pramipexole and ropinirole). Treatment of ICDs requires reduction, and usually elimination of the offending medication. Since the ICD behaviours may not be immediately associated with treatment by the patient, and because they may be perceived as socially undesirable, it is important for the physician to counsel patients about ICDs prior to starting treatment with a dopamine agonist.

Sleep. Patients with PD have a range of sleep problems. The most common of these are insomnia and excessive daytime sleepiness. Patients with insomnia usually are able to fall asleep, but awaken in the middle of the night and are unable to fall asleep again. In some cases, this problem is made worse by night-time wearing-off of dopaminergic medications. Poor sleep may also be related to nocturia or underlying depression.

Excessive daytime sleepiness occurs frequently and may result from poor sleep at night, sedating effects of dopaminergic medications or decreased alertness directly attributable to PD pathology. Relative hypotension, particularly early in the morning and after meals, may contribute to daytime drowsiness. Again, careful history taking can help to identify the specific cause of drowsiness.

REM sleep behaviour disorder (RBD) is a parasomnia that is highly associated with PD, and RBD symptoms may precede the onset of motor symptoms of PD by a number of years. RBD may manifest as thrashing, falling out of bed, calling out, or hitting the bed-partner during sleep. Injury to the patient or bed partner can occur.

Autonomic. The involvement of the autonomic nervous system PD in PD is variable and may result in a range of gastro-intestinal, genitourinary, and circulatory symptoms.

Constipation is the most common gastro-intestinal symptom. If untreated, it can result in fecal impaction and avoidable visits to the emergency room. Weight loss may occur due to reduced food intake and is compounded by the increased energy expenditure incurred by rigidity and/or dyskinesias. Dental and salivary problems, swallowing difficulties and impaired gastric emptying also contribute to weight loss. Delayed gastric emptying is common and contributes to erratic response to dopaminergic medications.

Urinary dysfunction is characterized by urgency and frequency. Nocturia is particularly common in men. Urinary incontinence is a very bothersome problem in patients with advanced PD. Impaired mobility may complicate urinary incontinence by making it more difficult to reach the bathroom in a timely fashion. Sexual dysfunction results from impotence, depression, and general physical disability.

Orthostatic hypotension may complicate typical PD, but is more common in multiple systems atrophy (MSA). Orthostasis may present as lightheadedness with standing or more subtle problems such as difficulty with concentration or headache. It may be partially responsible for the transient reductions in alertness that affect patients with advanced PD and dementia. Orthostasis tends to be most severe early in the morning and after meals. Medications used to treat PD, including dopaminergic and anti-cholinergic medications, can exacerbate hypotension. A drug history is important in the evaluation of orthostatis, since many patients may have been left on traditional anti-hypertensive medications in spite of below-normal blood pressure. Treatment for orthostatis includes non-pharmacological measures such as compression stockings and liberalization of salt intake. Medications to increase blood pressure including fludrocortisone and midodrine may be used if needed.

Sensory. Sensory symptoms in PD are increasingly recognized as a frequent and disabling complaint. Patients may report numbness, paresthesias, burning, itching, or crawling, associated with their PD. In some cases, these symptoms fluctuate with respect to dopaminergic replacement therapy. Restlessness, internal tremulousness, shooting sensations, and muscle aches are common. Pain in PD is multifactorial. The rigidity and slowness of PD inevitably cause discomfort via cramping, arthritis, postural changes and contractures. However, there is evidence to suggest that a primary, central-type of PD pain contributes as well.

Olfactory dysfunction is an early and common manifestation of PD. Degree of smell loss is only modestly associated severity of other features of PD, may precede detectable motor symptoms, and is not affected by dopaminergic treatment.

Visual problems can occur in PD. Loss of acuity, blurring, impaired near vision with convergence insufficiency, abnormal color discrimination, and abnormal light sensitivity have been described. Patients also may report problems reading, specifically describing difficulty following across the line of text.

3.4 **Summary**

PD is primarily characterized by the motor features of tremor rigidity and bradykinesia. These problems progress over time and treatment-related motor complications may also develop with disease progression. Non-motor problems, particularly dementia, but also a Pandora's box of other features, complicate the middle and later stages of PD and contribute substantially to overall disability.

References and further reading

Emre M. (2003) Dementia associated with Parkinson's disease. *Lancet Neurology*, **2**, 229–37.

Friedman J.H. and Chou K.L. (2004) Sleep and fatigue in Parkinson's disease. *Parkinsonism and Related Disorders*, **10**, S27–S35.

Hely M.A., Morris J.G., Reid W.G., Trafficante R. (2005) Sydney Multicenter Study of Parkinson's disease: non-L-dopa-responsive problems dominate at 15 years. *Mov Disord*, **20**, 190–9.

Miyasaki J.M., Shannon K., Voon V., Ravina B., Kleiner-Fisman G., Anderson K. *et al.* (2006) Practice Parameter: evaluation and treatment of depression, psychosis, and dementia in Parkinson disease (an evidence-based review): report of the Quality Standards Subcommittee of the American Academy of Neurology. *Neurology*, **66**, 996–1002.

Paulson H.L., Stern M.B. (2004) Clinical manifestations of Parkinson's disease. In: Watts R.L., Koller W.C., eds. *Movement Disorders: Neurological Principles and Practice*. New York: McGraw-Hill, 223–46.

Suchowersky O., Reich S., Perlmutter J., Zesiewica T., Gronseth G., Weiner W.J. (2006) Practice parameter: Diagnosis and prognosis of new onset Parkinson disease (an evidence-based review): Report of the Quality Standards Subcommittee of the American Academy of Neurology. *Neurology*, **66**, 968–75.

van Dijk J.G., Haan J., Zwinderman K., Kremer B., van Hilten B.J., Roos R.A. (1993) Autonomic nervous system dysfunction in Parkinson's disease: relationships with age, medication, duration, and severity. *J Neurol Neurosurg Psychiatry*, **56**, 1090–5.

Chapter 4

Differential diagnosis

Bryan T. Klaasen and Charles H. Adler

Key points

- The differential diagnosis of Parkinson's disease includes other neurodegenerative diseases as well as potentially treatable secondary conditions
- A thorough medication history should be obtained for all patients presenting with parkinsonism
- Wilson's disease should be considered in all patients under the age of 50
- Treatment with dopaminergic medications should be considered for all patients with parkinsonism as benefit may be seen even for some secondary causes.

Parkinson's disease (PD) refers to the specific condition of Lewy body positive neuronal degeneration within the substantia nigra, while parkinsonism refers to the clinical syndrome of rest tremor, rigidity, bradykinesia, and postural instability that can result from a variety of pathophysiologic insults. Because some causes of parkinsonism are specifically treatable, it is important to have a solid understanding of the differential diagnosis of PD.

4.1 Symptomatic parkinsonism

4.1.1 Drug-induced parkinsonism

As drug-induced parkinsonism is usually easily treated by withdrawal of the offending agent, a careful medication history should be elicited from every patient presenting with parkinsonian signs. Clues suggesting drug-induced parkinsonism include a subacute onset of symmetric symptoms, early presence of postural tremor, and oral-buccal dyskinesias; however, in some cases the presentation is indistinguishable from that of idiopathic PD.

Dopamine receptor blocking agents (neuroleptics) with a high affinity for the D2 dopamine receptor are the most common culprits. It should be remembered that these mediations are used not only for psychosis but also for nausea and vomiting. Drugs of several other medication classes have also been reported to cause parkinsonian signs and are listed in Table 4.1.

Table 4.1 Medications with potential to cause or exacerbate parkinsonism	
Dopamine receptor blocking agents (neuroleptics)	**Dopamine depleting agents**
Butyrophenones	alpha-Methyldopa
Haloperidol	Reserpine
Droperidol	Tetrabenazine
Phenothiazines	**Calcium channel blockers**
Chlorpromazine	Cinnarizine
Fluphenazine	Flunarizine
Mesoridazine	Diltiazem
Perphenazine	Verapamil
Prochlorperazine	**Other medications**
Promazine	Amiodarone
Promethazine	Amphotericin B
Thiethylperazine	Bethanechol
Thioridazine	Captopril
Trifluoperazine	Ciclosporin
Thioxanthenes	Cyclophosphamide
Chlorprothixene	Cytarabine
Flupentixol	Diazepam
Thiothixene	Fluoxetine and other SSRIs
Substituted benzamides	Lithium
Cisapride	Lovastatin
Domperidone	Meperidine
Metoclopramide	Phenelzine
'Atypical antipsychotic agents'	Phenytoin
Clozapine	Procaine
Loxapine	Pyridostigmine
Olanzapine	Tacrine
Risperidone	Valproic acid
Quetiapine	
Ziprasidone	

Initial treatment of drug-induced parkinsonism is withdrawal of the offending agent, if possible. While this iatrogenic condition is typically reversible, resolution of symptoms can be prolonged, taking from six to 12 months in some cases. If the offending agent cannot be discontinued then one must consider the safety of treating with dopaminergic medications and/or amantadine. If parkinsonism does not resolve with drug withdrawal then it is possible the drug unmasked the patient's predisposition for developing PD.

4.1.2 Toxin-induced parkinsonism

Exposure to toxins causing selective damage to the substantia nigra or basal ganglia can potentially result in irreversible parkinsonism. These agents are often used in the laboratory to create animal models of PD. The most notorious of these, a byproduct of meperidine synthesis known as MPTP, selectively destroys nigral neurons and caused several cases of parkinsonism affecting drug abusers in the early 1980s. No recent cases of MPTP-induced parkinsonism have been reported.

Manganese toxicity can result in parkinsonism, though rest tremor is rare and there is often an associated dystonia. Those at risk for manganese toxicity include manganese miners, welders, and intravenous methcathinone (ephedrone) users in Eastern Europe and Russia. MR imaging shows increased T1 signal in the bilateral globus pallidus, and chelation therapy may be of benefit to some patients.

Hypoxia induced by carbon monoxide poisoning can cause bilateral globus pallidus necrosis and subsequent parkinsonism; however, most of these patients have more widespread deficits due to the profound hypoxia. Acute or chronic cyanide exposure not leading to death can cause parkinsonism, possibly secondary to necrosis of the globus pallidus, putamen, and subthalamic nucleus. Herbicides, such as diquat or paraquat, that are chemically related to MPTP have been associated with a parkinsonian syndrome as have organophosphate pesticides. Industrial chemicals including carbon disulfide, methanol, n-hexane, and lacquer thinner have also been reported to cause parkinsonism.

4.1.3 Vascular parkinsonism

Acute ischemic infarction of the caudate, putamen, globus pallidus, or brain stem can result in parkinsonism. The diagnosis is based on the abrupt onset of symptoms with step-wise progression in a patient with vascular risk factors such as hypertension or diabetes. Other neurologic signs such as aphasia or corticospinal tract dysfunction are often present. Brain MR imaging may reveal the causative lesion; however, the presence of a basal ganglia infarction on neuroimaging is not sufficient to make a diagnosis of vascular parkinsonism given the frequency of this finding in the general population.

4.1.4 **Structural lesions**

Mass lesions of the midbrain, basal ganglia, or ventricular outflow pathways are an uncommon cause of parkinsonism. Causative lesions include tumor, abscess, aneurysm, or hematoma (including subdural hematoma). In most cases there are other associated neurologic signs that would prompt the clinician to order a neuroimaging study showing the lesion.

4.1.5 **Hydrocephalus**

Hydrocephalus results from increased CSF production or impairment of CSF outflow; this can be secondary to obstruction within the ventricular system (obstructive hydrocephalus) or poor CSF absorption back into the venous system (communicating hydrocephalus). Parkinsonism has rarely been reported as a feature of obstructive hydrocephalus. Those with communicating hydrocephalus can develop the syndrome of normal pressure hydrocephalus (NPH), in which gait dysfunction, cognitive decline, and urinary incontinence are the predominant features. The gait disorder has parkinsonian features such as flexed posture with slow, shuffling steps. However, NPH patients often have a wide-based gait and relative sparing of the upper body which can help to differentiate them from those with idiopathic PD. Symptoms from both obstructive and communicating hydrocephalus may respond to ventriculoperitoneal shunting.

4.1.6 **Infections**

In the first half of the 20th century, cases of parkinsonism developing after encephalitis lethargica were common. Postencephalitic parkinsonism occurred predominantly in the teens and twenties and could develop acutely with the encephalitis or insidiously many years after the event. In the current era, this condition has rarely been reported. Fungal infections that cause a mass lesion may result in parkinsonism.

Creutzfeldt-Jakob disease is a prion disease presenting as a rapidly progressive neurodegenerative syndrome. While the clinical picture is dominated by dementia, other neurologic features such as ataxia, myoclonus, and parkinsonism can be present. The rapid course and associated symptoms should distinguish this disorder from Parkinson's disease.

Patients with HIV can develop parkinsonism in isolation or in company with HIV-associated dementia. HIV-infected patients are also more likely to develop drug-induced parkinsonism in the presence of an offending agent.

4.1.7 **Acquired metabolic**

Hypothyroidism can result in generalized bradykinesia, ataxia, and tremor which might be mistaken for mild parkinsonism. More specific signs of PD such as dampened amplitude of alternating motion rate, cogwheel rigidity, and the typical parkinsonian tremor and gait are usually absent. However, as the condition is easily treated with thyroid hormone replacement, it is reasonable to check thyroid studies as a part of the initial evaluation of parkinsonism.

Hypoparathyroidism can result in basal ganglia calcification and subsequent parkinsonism. Hyperparathyroidism can worsen the symptoms of pre-existent PD. Evaluating the serum calcium level is an adequate screening for either condition.

4.1.8 Posttraumatic

Repeated concussive head injury, such as experienced by boxers, can result in parkinsonism, ataxia, dementia, and personality changes. The constellation has been termed *dementia pugilistica*. Only rarely have single, severe head injuries been associated with parkinsonism. Though some epidemiologic studies have found a correlation between remote minor head trauma and PD, its importance as a risk factor remains unclear.

4.1.9 Hemiatrophy-hemiparkinsonism

Patients with the rare hemiatrophy-hemiparkinsonism syndrome usually have atrophy of one side of the body present from childhood. Ipsilateral parkinsonism develops years later and can be associated with dystonia. Contralateral brain atrophy is often present on neuroimaging. Many of these patients have a favorable response to levodopa.

4.2 Neurodegenerative disorders associated with parkinsonism

4.2.1 Progressive supranuclear palsy

Progressive supranuclear palsy (PSP) is commonly misdiagnosed as PD early in the course of illness. The initial presentation as an akinetic-rigid syndrome may be indistinguishable from PD. However, in PSP rest tremor is rare, axial rigidity is usually greater than appendicular rigidity, kyphosis is minimal, and postural instability occurs early in the disease course. Patients with PSP often have a characteristic facial expression with a wide eyed, worried look. The supranuclear opthalmoparesis is typically most severe with downgaze, and impaired vertical saccades may be an even earlier sign. Pseudobulbar symptoms such as dysarthria, dysphagia, and uncontrolled crying or laughing are more commonly seen in PSP than PD.

Midbrain atrophy is the classic finding on MR but is not appreciated in all cases. The course of PSP is more aggressive than that of PD. Patients often have a response to dopaminergic treatment initially, but this is rarely sustained.

4.2.2 **Multiple system atrophy**

Multiple system atrophy is a multi-level neurodegenerative condition with predominantly parkinsonian (MSA-P), cerebellar (MSA-C), and dysautonomic (MSA-A) presentations. MSA-P, formerly termed striatonigral degeneration, presents as parkinsonism without tremor. Cerebellar, autonomic, and corticospinal tract findings are usually present to some degree and can be clinical clues to the diagnosis. As in PSP, prominent postural instability with early falls is common in MSA-P. Nocturnal stridor is present in MSA and can be a helpful diagnostic clue; this symptom must be closely monitored as potentially fatal airway obstruction can result.

MR imaging may show abnormalities of the brain stem, cerebellum, or striatum. Progression in MSA is more rapid than in PD. As with PSP, patients have a variable response to dopaminergic treatment initially that is not sustained long-term.

4.2.3 **Dementia with Lewy bodies**

Dementia with Lewy bodies (DLB) is characterized by progressive dementia, fluctuations in cognitive function, well-formed visual hallucinations, and parkinsonism. In contrast to the later onset of cognitive decline and dementia in PD, early cognitive dysfunction is seen in DLB. Cognitive decline must precede or occur within one year of motor findings for a clinical diagnosis of DLB to be made. In DLB, rest tremor is present less often and myoclonus more often than in PD. Syncope, repeated falls, and neuroleptic sensitivity are associated features in DLB.

The pathology of DLB and PD differs mainly in distribution, with a greater cortical and limbic burden of Lewy bodies being present in DLB. Additionally, most cases of DLB also meet pathologic criteria for co-existent Alzheimer's disease. Treatment of the motor symptoms can be difficult because dopaminergic agents often worsen the hallucinations.

4.2.4 **Alzheimer's disease**

A substantial proportion of patients with Alzheimer's type dementia have associated parkinsonism. Rigidity, bradykinesia, and gait disorder can all be present but are usually a minor component of the overall clinical syndrome. Rest tremor is rare. Cognitive difficulties usually precede motor symptoms by many years.

It is important to note that PD itself is associated with a subcortical dementia. Neuropsychometric testing may help to differentiate between the cognitive decline associated with PD versus AD. However, the most helpful clue to diagnosis is the symptom course: motor symptoms that precede cognitive decline by years are more consistent with PD while AD and DLB have cognitive decline as a presenting or co-existent feature at onset of motor decline.

4.2.5 Corticobasal degeneration

Classically presenting as a progressive, markedly asymmetric rigidity and apraxia, corticobasal degeneration (CBD) can also include tremor, bradykinesia, and postural instability. The involved limb (usually an arm) is often held in a fixed, dystonic posture with wrist flexed and fingers extended. Features in common with the atypical parkinsonian syndromes include hyperreflexia, pseudobulbar palsy, and supranuclear gaze palsy. Cortical sensory loss and myoclonus can be present. In some cases, the affected limb moves involuntarily and the patient does not recognize it as his or her own, the so-called alien-limb phenomena. While this is quite helpful in differentiating CBD from other parkinsonian syndromes, the alien-limb phenomenon is not present in all cases.

MR imaging may demonstrate asymmetry of parietal sulci with marked atrophy on the side contralateral to the affected limb. CBD is not levodopa responsive.

4.3 Hereditary disorders associated with parkinsonism

4.3.1 Wilson's disease

Wilson's disease is a rare, autosomal-recessive inborn error of metabolism presenting in the second and third decades and resulting in deficient biliary excretion of copper. The ensuing systemic copper overload results in tissue deposition initially confined to the liver causing hepatitis or hepatic failure. When the storage capacity of the liver is overwhelmed, copper can overflow into the central nervous system with a predilection for deposition within the basal ganglia. In 40% of patients, neurologic symptoms precede symptoms of hepatic disease. Motor symptoms can include resting or action tremor, dysarthria, slowed saccades, dystonia, rigidity, and bradykinesia. Cognitive decline and psychiatric symptoms including depression, mania, personality change, and psychosis are frequent features of the disease. Because of the heterogeneity of presentation and the potential for treatment, Wilson's disease should be considered in any patient under the age of 50 presenting with a movement disorder.

The diagnosis can be made by finding low levels of serum ceruloplasmin, high 24 hour urinary copper excretion, and Kayser-Fleischer rings on slit-lamp examination. If these tests are inconclusive, liver biopsy with quantification of hepatic copper content is the gold standard for diagnosis. Treatment includes reduction of dietary copper and chelation with penicillamine, trientine, or zinc. Ammonium tetrathiomolybdate, which blocks copper absorption, has also been used with some success.

4.3.2 **Huntington's disease**

Huntington's disease (HD) is an autosomal-dominant trinucelotide repeat disorder. Cognitive and neuropsychiatric problems are often the earliest signs. Though the motor manifestations are classically characterized by chorea, HD can present as a mainly bradykinetic disorder in those under age 20 and rarely in adults. Patients may respond to levodopa. The possibility of HD should be considered in the evaluation of juvenile parkinsonism.

4.3.3 **Dopa responsive dystonia**

Dopa responsive dystonia, an inherited condition of deficient catecholamine synthesis, can present with parkinsonism in addition to dystonia. The onset is usually in childhood, and as the name implies, both the dystonia and parkinsonism are exquisitely responsive to levodopa therapy.

4.3.4 **Rapid-onset dystonia-parkinsonism**

Rapid-onset dystonia-parkinsonism is an autosomal-dominant condition in which affected individuals have the onset of dystonia and parkinsonism over hours to days. Symptoms usually stabilize within a few weeks, after which there is no or only slow progression. The disease is characterized by a poor levodopa response. Mutations in the alpha-3 subunit of the Na-K-ATPase have been found in patients with the disorder.

4.3.5 **X-linked dystonia-parkinsonism (Lubag)**

Lubag is an X-linked recessive disorder of Filipino males that can present with either parkinsonism or dystonia. Patients initially presenting with dystonia inevitably develop parkinsonism as the disease progresses; however, some patients presenting with parkinsonism maintain a chiefly parkinsonian phenotype. Treatment is usually only modestly effective.

4.3.6 **Dentatorubral-pallidoluysian atrophy**

Dentatorubral-pallidoluysian atrophy (DRPLA) is a rare autosomal dominant trinucleotide repeat disorder with age of onset from childhood to late adult life. There is wide phenotypic expression including bradykinesia, rigidity, and tremor along with choreoathetosis, dystonia, ataxia, and myoclonus. Dementia and psychiatric symptoms can be prominent features. Because the parkinsonian signs rarely occur in isolation, DRPLA is more likely to be confused with HD than PD.

4.3.7 **Spinocerebellar ataxia type 3 (Machado-Joseph disease)**

The clinical spectrum of the spinocerebellar ataxias (SCA) may includ parkinsonism, and this is especially the case for SCA-3 (Machad Joseph disease), an autosomal dominant trinucleotide repeat disor

In addition to parkinsonism, clinical features can include cerebellar ataxia, supranuclear opthalmoplegia, dysphagia, dystonia, hyperreflexia, and amyotrophy. Though parkinsonism can be the predominant feature, it rarely occurs in isolation and SCA-3 is therefore more likely to be confused with MSA than PD.

4.4 **Other disorders**

4.4.1 **Essential tremor**

Essential tremor (ET) is a condition commonly confused with PD despite its distinguishing characteristics (Table 4.2). ET most often presents as a symmetric postural and action tremor that resolves with rest. Because of possible overlap of tremor phenomenology, the best way to distinguish ET from PD is the former's lack of bradykinesia, rigidity, gait disorder, and postural instability as well as its poor dopamine response.

4.4.2 **Psychogenic parkinsonism**

As is the case for most other movement disorders, psychogenic variants of parkinsonism exist. Clues to suggest a psychogenic cause include an abrupt onset of severe symptoms, static course, and spontaneous remission. The tremor frequency and amplitude can be variable, and both tremor and rigidity are often distractible. Rapid alternating movements are deliberate and irregular but often sustainable without the typical dampening of amplitude seen in PD. The gait exam may show findings not typical for PD. However, as with all psychogenic disorders, psychogenic parkinsonism remains a diagnosis of exclusion and an appropriate diagnostic workup should be arranged.

Table 4.2 Clinical features of essential tremor and Parkinson's disease

Essential tremor	Parkinson's disease
Tremor with posture and action (May have rest tremor in advanced disease)	Tremor at rest (May have associated postural or action tremor)
6–12 Hz	4–7 Hz
Bilateral and symmetric	Asymmetric
Head and vocal tremor	Mouth, jaw, and leg tremor

References and further reading

Cordato N. J., Halliday G. M., Caine D. & Morris J. G. (2006) Comparison of motor, cognitive, and behavioral features in progressive supranuclear palsy and Parkinson's disease. *Mov Disord.* **21,** 632–8.

Dobyns W. B., Ozelius L. J., Kramer P. L., Brashear A., Farlow M. R., Perry T. R., Walsh L. E., Kasarskis E. J., Butler I. J. & Breakefield X. O. (1993) Rapid-onset dystonia-parkinsonism. *Neurology* **43,** 2596–602.

Evidente V. G., Gwinn-Hardy K., Hardy,J., Hernandez D. & Singleton A. (2002) X-linked dystonia ('Lubag') presenting predominantly with parkinsonism: a more benign phenotype? *Mov Disord.* **17,** 200–2.

Kollensperger M., Geser F., Seppi K., Stampfer-Kountchev M., Sawires M., Scherfler C., Boesch S., Mueller J., Koukouni V., Quinn N., Pellecchia M. T., Barone P., Schimke N., Dodel R., Oertel W., Dupont E., Ostergaard K., Daniels C., Deuschl G., Gurevich T., Giladi N., Coelho M., Sampaio C., Nilsson C., Widner H., Sorbo F. D., Albanese A., Cardozo A., Tolosa E., Abele M., Klockgether T., Kamm C., Gasser T., Djaldetti R., Colosimo C., Meco G., Schrag A., Poewe W. & Wenning G. K. (2008) Red flags for multiple system atrophy. *Mov Disord.* **23,** 1093–9.

Machado A., Chien H. F., Deguti M. M., Cancado E., Azevedo R. S., Scaff M. & Barbosa E. R. (2006) Neurological manifestations in Wilson's disease: Report of 119 cases. *Mov Disord.* **21,** 2192–6.

Mckeith I. G., Dickson D. W., Lowe J., Emre M., O'brien J. T., Feldman H., Cummings J., Duda J. E., Lippa C., Perry E. K., Aarsland D., Arai H., Ballard C. G., Boeve B., Burn D. J., Costa D., Del Ser T., Dubois B., Galasko D., Gauthier S., Goetz C. G., Gomez-Tortosa E., Halliday G., Hansen L. A., Hardy J., Iwatsubo T., Kalaria R. N., Kaufer D., Kenny R. A., Korczyn A., Kosaka K., Lee V. M., Lees A., Litvan I., Londos E., Lopez O. L., Minoshima S., Mizuno Y., MolinaJ. A., Mukaetova-Ladinska E. B., Pasquier F., Perry R. H., Schulz J. B., Trojanowski J. Q. & Yamada M. (2005) Diagnosis and management of dementia with Lewy bodies: third report of the DLB Consortium. *Neurology* **65,** 1863–72.

Nahab F. B., Peckham E. & Hallett M. (2007) Essential tremor, deceptively simple. *Pract Neurol.* **7,** 222–33.

Stepens A., Logina I., Liguts V., Aldins P., Eksteina I., Platkajis A., Martinsone I., Terauds E., Rozentale B. & Donaghy M. (2008) A Parkinsonian syndrome in methcathinone users and the role of manganese. *N Engl J Med.* **358,** 1009–17.

Tse W., Cersosimo M.G., Gracies J. M., Morgello S., Olanow C. W. & Koller W. (2004) Movement disorders and AIDS: a review. *Parkinsonism Relat Disord.* **10,** 323–34.

Van Gerpen J. A. (2002) Drug-induced parkinsonism. *Neurologist,* **8,** 363–70.

Wijemanne S. & Jankovic J. (2007) Hemiparkinsonism-hemiatrophy syndrome. *Neurology,* **69,** 1585–94.

Zijlmans J. C., Daniel S. E., Hughes A. J., Revesz T. & Lees A. J. (2004) Clinicopathological investigation of vascular parkinsonism, including clinical criteria for diagnosis. *Mov Disord.* **19,** 630–40.

Chapter 5

Imaging

Nico L. Leenders

Key points

- Neuroimaging by itself can not establish a diagnosis of Parkinson's Disease (PD) or related disorders. However, in the appropriate clinical context it can provide key information
- MRI or CT scans are useful in excluding comorbidity or proving alternative causes of parkinsonisms, but do not contribute to making a diagnosis of PD
- Dopaminergic radiotracers as used in SPECT and PET brain scanning are extremely useful within the right clinical context, but need to be applied and interpreted with caution
- Cerebral glucose metabolism as measured using PET scanning can be applied usefully in neurodegenerative brain diseases to guide the clinician in the complex field of parkinsonian conditions or dementias
- Sonography is a promising method which may obtain a place in early diagnosis of PD, but overlap with healthy controls and other conditions can be considerable and in a fairly large number of subjects it is not possible to obtain an adequate acoustical window.

5.1 Introduction

The diagnosis of Parkinson's disease (PD) is based primarily on clinical grounds. A patient who presents with typical signs and symptoms and responds favourably and easily to common drug regimens does not need any neuroimaging investigation to underscore the diagnosis. However, in practice physicians are confronted regularly with patients whose medical history contains puzzling elements or who show signs and symptoms of parkinsonism but with uncommon features or whose clinical condition is too mild to be sure of a diagnosis. Within that complexity neuroimaging with either 'structural' or 'functional' information can be very useful.

In general, it can be said that in daily practice brain scans are requested much more often than strictly speaking is necessary. It must be stated here that an image of the brain hardly ever proves a diagnosis in the field of brain degeneration like PD and related disorders. Thus an image of the brain in that clinical context is not proof of a disease and therefore a report of, e.g. a SPECT or PET scan illustrating striatal uptake of a dopaminergic tracer cannot state that the investigated subject has PD or not. The report of such a scan can only indicate whether the biochemical activity underlying the processing of the applied tracer is normal or abnormal and in which brain regions. The interpretation of that finding will depend entirely on the pertinent clinical picture. Sometimes a combination of several neuroimaging methods will be necessary to provide the correct conclusion or follow-up lasting for years may be required before a patient's condition becomes clear. In this chapter only the perceived established facts concerning neuroimaging in PD will be summarized. Much of the detail is available in the literature and new methods are continuously being developed and tried, but before a new method is sufficiently validated in clinical practice a long and cumbersome path has normally to be followed.

When neuroimaging is applied a distinction is usually made between 'structural' and 'functional' methods. The first relate mostly to MRI or CT scans and the latter, e.g. to radiotracer studies. Such a distinction is rather artificial and it is preferable to state the specific information which is sought and then to determine which scanning method is appropriate. Is it a specific biochemical activity at certain locations in the brain which is of interest, or is it necessary to receive information about, for example, white matter vascular lesions? Also, sonography is referred to as 'structural' neuroimaging method even though the method is based on the echogenicity of brain tissue from which the 'structure' of some regions are being inferred. For convenience, however, the scanning methods which are performed in patients with PD are discussed briefly below according to common practice.

5.2 CT/MRI

5.2.1 General information

MRI and CT scans can provide excellent information about disease conditions which are not related to PD, but which may give rise to secondary parkinsonism or might explain coincidental comorbidity existing in addition to PD.

For instance, normal pressure hydrocephalus can be suspected or multi-infarcts can be shown. Also, rarer cases can be shown when, e.g. a brain tumor patient or an unexpected juvenile Huntington's disease patient presents with parkinsonism, discovered by abnormalities on a MRI or CT scan. There is discussion as to whether a CT or MRI scan should be performed in all new cases with parkinsonism in order to systematically exclude or confirm secondary parkinsonism or comorbidity even if the classical signs and symptoms of PD are present.

5.2.2 **Specific information**

Neurodegenerative brain diseases like Alzheimer's disease (AD) or PD are generally accompanied by global atrophy of the brain particularly at the later stages. But these findings are neither helpful in making a diagnosis nor in distinguishing the various conditions from each other. In some instances at later stages the accentuation of regional atrophy may support a certain diagnosis, e.g. frontotemporal dementia or corticobasal degeneration (CBD), but at that stage the diagnosis usually has already become clear on clinical grounds. The same is true for some more specific alterations in some diseases in which parkinsonism may be an important feature. In MSA, e.g. typical signal increases can be seen in T2 weighted MRI images at the level of brain stem ('hot cross bun sign', atrophy of medial cerebellar peduncle) or basal ganglia ('putaminal ridge') and others. If found this is almost pathognomonic. However, it is not always present and then only late in the development of the disease. In a PSP patient the superior cerebellar peduncle is especially atrophic giving rise to a smaller mesencephalon (sometimes in a sagittal view seen as a 'humming bird' sign) and also other changes can be found like atrophic corpus callosum. However, to determine these changes it is necessary to have the scans taken in a protocol led way and measure in a standard fashion the various sizes of the targeted brain regions. These measures have then to be compared with normal values. Such a procedure is, however, seldom done in clinical radiological practice. Other specific information is seen occasionally in rare cases of PKAN (pantothenate kinase associated neurodegeneration. Abnormal iron accumulation in various brain nuclei such as globus pallidus plus central necrosis: 'eye of the tiger' sign) or Wilson's disease (increased T2 MRI signals in lenticular nuclei, thalami, and other regions). Although these conditions normally present with different signs and symptoms, parkinsonism may sometimes be a presenting sign. PD patients do not show any specific changes on their CT of MRI scans. Here it may be stated that the terms 'variant', 'atypical' PD, or 'Parkinson plus' when indicating, e.g. MSA or PSP are misnomers which confuse the thinking about PD, and these terms should be avoided. Indeed, variants of PD do exist (like tremor dominant PD, monogenetic variant of PD, Parkinson's disease with dementia (PDD), or dementia with Lewy bodies (DLB)), but MSA, PSP, CBD and others are different diseases.

5.3 Radiotracer imaging (PET and SPECT)

5.3.1 General comments

Using these methods one needs to consider what is actually being measured. Just stating that 'a PET scan or a SPECT has been done' is meaningless. It is preferable to state the name of the applied radiotracer since this relates directly to the core information obtained, namely a specific regional biochemical activity. Thinking about the meaning of the measurement is thereby guided more easily. There are no fundamental differences between PET and SPECT scanning techniques since both measure gamma rays emanating from the body after a radiotracer has been administered (usually intravenously). Both methods assess the location and intensity of the radiotracer on the basis of the collected gamma rays during the scan. Gamma rays are high energy electromagnetic waves emitted from the nucleus of a decaying atom, the unstable isotope of the stable parent form. The tracer compound is by definition radio-labelled with these isotopes in order to indicate where the tracer is located at a certain time point. The used isotopes are unstable forms of, e.g. carbon, fluor in the case of PET radiotracers and technetium, or iodine in the case of SPECT radiotracers. Since the accumulation of the tracer is dependent on the local biochemical trapping of the tracer or its metabolized product the assessed intensity of radioactivity relates directly to the specific biochemical property of the tracer compound.

However, there are a number of practical differences between PET and SPECT. Some will be named here. PET radiotracers are labelled with isotopes which decay by emitting a positron from its nucleus which then almost immediately is converted into two simultaneous gamma rays moving into opposite directions. This allows a high sensitivity recovering the signals from the tissue and makes quantification easier. Also the use of physiological radiolabels (carbon-11 or fluor-18) allows many compounds to be labelled without altering their property. The radioactive half-life is short for these isotopes (minutes rather than hours) which allows dynamic biochemichal processes to be studied. On the other hand, the production of short-lived radiotracers requires an accelerator and sophisticated radiochemical laboratory on site. Also, for clinical practice the property of exact quantification is not always necessary and relative uptake values may be of sufficient value.

SPECT radiotracers have a much longer half-life and can be produced centrally and distributed commercially over many centres. The radiolabels are either non-physiological or large in size and thereby alter the compound properties. However, this may not be a problem if the properties of the tracer are well characterized. Since the SPECT isotopes decay emitting only one gamma ray ('single photon') it is more difficult with this scanning method to assess from which location the signal is coming.

The availability of SPECT scans is currently much larger than that of PET. However, since FDG is increasingly being produced commercially (half-life almost two hours) and being provided to many nuclear medicine departments for whole body oncology scans, the availability of FDG PET scans for brain studies is increasing rapidly.

5.3.2 PET (positron emission tomography)

5.3.2.1 *Dopaminergic tracers*

FDOPA (dihydroxyphenylalanin labeled with fluor-18) was the first radiotracer being developed to trace the biochemical dopaminergic properties of brain regions using PET scans. FDOPA is being decarboxylated or methylated, like endogenous L-dopa or the therapeutically administered levodopa in PD patients. First this takes place peripherally in the blood resulting in F-dopamine or F-methyldopa. The amine does not pass the blood-brain barrier (BBB), but F-dopa and F-methyldopa do enter the brain. In order to inhibit peripheral dopa-decarboxylase usually carbidopa (1mg/kg body weight) is given orally one hour before administering FDOPA. This makes more FDOPA available for entering the brain and to provide the necessary counting statistics during the scanning. Surprisingly the second peripheral metabolic pathway (methylation) is normally not being blocked although this would provide a further considerable increase in FDOPA availability to the brain. Approved drugs like entacapone or tolcapone could be applied. The safe use of the combined blockage has been shown experimentally by various groups. It would also increase the contrast between uptake of FDOPA in the target regions and the rest of the brain since it would avoid non-specific brain uptake of F-methylated dopa.

When FDOPA enters the brain it will partly be taken up by the nerve terminals of the predominant nigrostriatal dopaminergic neurons, decarboxylated into F-dopamine and to some extent be accumulated there. Essential in this process is the trapping part of the enzymatic product namely F-dopamine. This allows assessment of the integrity of the dopaminergic nerve terminals in comparison to non-target reference regions of the brain or (in more research settings) in comparison to the peripheral blood activity representing the delivery of the tracer to the brain. Thus specific striatal uptake after intravenous FDOPA administration indicates mainly the biochemical activity of local dopa-decarboxylase.

In PD one of the important pathological features is the degeneration of part of the dopaminergic neurons in the substantia nigra (SN). This has also consequences for the projection neurons which mainly terminate in the striatum. Since in PD the lateral part of the SN

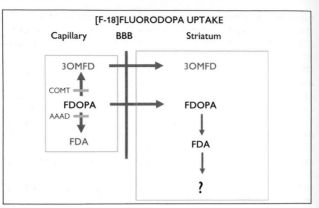

Figure 5.1 Schematic drawing of FDOPA uptake into striatum (see text).
BBB = Blood-brain barrier. COMT = CO-methyltransferase. AAAD = aromatic
amino acid decarboxylase. 3OMFD = 3O-methyl-fluorodopa. FDA = fluorodopamine.

degenerates first the reduced activity of dopa-decarboxylase at the
striatal level occurs first in the dorsal parts of the putamen. Because
of the location of the specific tracer uptake the FDOPA tracer is
sometimes called a 'presynaptic' tracer. At later stages other parts of
the putamen and even caudate nucleus may become affected. In the
affected striatal regions the activity of the enzyme dopadecarboxylase is diminished and thus less FDOPA can be converted into the
trapped product F-dopamine. Since the nerve terminals at early
stages are supposed to be still present (albeit with reduced enzyme
activity) the specific tracer conversion into F-dopamine can still be
trapped and thus be quantified or visualized. These reductions are
typically asymmetric in most PD patients and of course more pro-
nounced on the side contralaterally to the clinically more affected
side. However, sometimes the reverse is the case and this is not
explained so far if technical failures are excluded.

Although the disease may clinically appear to start on one side of
the body only, the specific FDOPA uptake may be reduced already
bilaterally also in the clinical unilateral cases. In fact the disease will
virtually always develop bilaterally clinically.

When the disease progresses the striatal tracer uptake defects will
become more severe and eventually show marked bilateral putaminal
defects (although initial asymmetries will usually prevail throughout
the disease course). However, there will almost always be a plateau
of remaining specific tracer uptake. This can easily be 25% of normal
values. Most likely this means that in PD the decline of the nigrostriatal
dopaminergic neuronal system is curvilinear (perhaps exponential).

Clinically this is reflected by the continuous positive response to levodopa substitution therapy in very late stages of the disease, although other negative features of the response pattern may have markedly reduced the quality of life.

It has been discussed frequently how soon a reduced striatal radiotracer uptake might discover a significant biochemical defect. It is speculated by extrapolation of cross-sectional data that the pathological reduction of striatal tracer uptake starts about 4 to 6 years before the diagnosis PD is made. Of course this does not mean that the disease PD itself starts at that point. Making an early diagnosis is important if one wishes to start symptomatic therapy early. An early radiotracer scan may help if the scan result is clearly pathological. However, if the result is doubtful then that should be clearly stated. Again a clinical diagnosis is made first on the basis of the clinical signs and symptoms. In the past few years various drug trials have been performed to test possible neuroprotection in PD. Striatal radiotracer uptake has been used in some of these to monitor disease progression. Unfortunately none of the proposed drugs were protective and thus no change of clinical time course or of altered tracer uptake was found.

A normal result of striatal FDOPA uptake should help to distinguish between a structural lesion of the dopaminergic nigrostriatal neurotransmitter system and other functional conditions like drug-induced (usually postsynaptically) parkinsonism, or rarely psychogenic parkinsonism. Other clinical conditions which are a mixture of beginning PD and another condition can be quite confusing and difficult to assess and requires a lot of experience.

Raclopride is a substance which binds to D2 dopamine receptors. In striatum these are preferentially located on the postsynaptic cell membrane and thus on the projection neurons originating from striatum and projecting to globus pallidus and substantia nigra. This substance can be radiolabelled with carbon-11 and its uptake into striatum measured using PET. It is also referred to as a 'postsynaptic' tracer. The tracer is not easy to produce radiochemically and not available in many centers and thus not often used in clinical practice. A reduction of tracer uptake in striatum can be found when the projection neurons are degenerating. That is not the case in PD and therefore normal values are generally being found. In some scientific studies comparing quantitative data using raclopride it can be seen that the postsynaptic receptor sites are initially and temporarily increased, or rather less intensely occupied by endogenous levodopa due to the diminished presynaptic delivery of neurotransmitter in PD. In other diseases like MSA or Huntington's chorea a local striatal reduction of tracer uptake can be found due to local striatal tissue loss. However, the easier tracer in this respect is FDG (see Section 5.3.2.2) which will give the same answer. When D2 receptor blocking drugs are being used by the patient the tracer uptake will then naturally be reduced.

Other dopaminergic tracers have been developed, but are either not validated or not widely available and thus not discussed here. Further developments will be in the field of scanners with higher resolution or sensitivity in order to investigate other regions of the brain, which so far have been too small or in which the binding sites are low in concentration thus requiring tracers with higher affinities. The consequences of these and other developments for clinical practice are as yet unclear.

5.3.2.2 *Glucose metabolism*

Cerebral glucose consumption can be measured by applying the radio-tracer FDG (fluorodeoxyglucose labeled with fluor-18) and PET (see Section 5.3.2). Currently there are no other tracers either for PET or for SPECT scanning available to measure glucose metabolism. The brain derives its energy from the oxidative metabolism of glucose and only in extreme conditions are other substances partly replacing glucose. The regional cerebral intensity of glucose metabolism reflects both the density of neuronal material (speak synapses) and its current activity. FDG will show the glucose metabolism of the whole brain and thus will give an immediate idea of which brain regions have altered energy consumption or in other words are pathologically altered. Usually reductions of metabolism are seen reflecting atrophy, infarcts and others. Only in some brain tumors or focal epileptic conditions can regional increases (sometimes remarkably so) be seen. It must be borne in mind that FDG uptake is the result of the accumulation of a metabolic product over many minutes and indicates a rather stable situation. It is normally in coupled balance with oxygen consumption and, to a certain, extent also with cerebral capillary blood flow. If one brain region is atrophic then all three measures will be usually to the same extent reduced. In contrast FDG brain uptake does not relate to the momentaneous changes in local oxygen consumption reflected by the BOLD signal as measured using functional MRI.

The fact that many brain degenerative diseases have a certain pattern of pathology in the brain can be demonstrated by many examples of altered in vivo patterns of FDG uptake. In classical cases of clearly developed clinical pictures the pattern can be discovered by the naked eye, but modern statistical image analysis can discern these patterns more reliably and in a more sophisticated way, particularly when the observer is unsure. Currently programs are being developed to compare the metabolic pattern of the individual patient with the various group specific disease patterns in order to detect as early as possible which neurodegenerative disease is at stake in each patient. It is suspected that in particular those patients who suffer from a

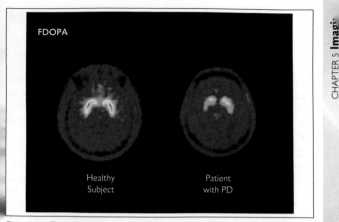

Figure 5.2 Typical transverse cross-sectional images of the brain after 45 minutes of application of the [F18] radiolabeled tracer fluorodopa (FDOPA). Intensity of uptake per picture element according to a linear color scale in which red represents the highest value and black the lowest. Top of the images is frontal and left-hand side of the image is the right side of the brain. The uptake in the central (striatal) regions of the brain is classically diminished in the patient with PD particularly in the posterior parts. In this patient the right posterior part of the striatum is most affected.

form of clinical parkinsonism with or without cognitive problems may benefit from this diagnostic process most. Idiopathic PD will usually not show dramatic changes in glucose metabolic patterns, but a relative prevalence of glucose use in striatum can often be seen. It is disputed whether this is the result of a global brain reduction with the exception e.g. of the striatum or whether the striatum in PD has locally increased metabolism. Other diseases accompanied by parkinsonism like MSA, PSP and others do show very different patterns. For example MSA patients have a clear local reduction of glucose use in striatal regions and PSP patients do show a typical medial frontal hypometabolism next to other regions. To study this complicated material the reader is referred to the published specialized literature.

5.3.3 SPECT (single photon emission computer tomography)

There exist many dopaminergic substances radiolabelled with a single photon emission isotope developed for use with SPECT. In practice however only two tracers are commonly used: FP-CIT and IBZM. FP-CIT has the same role in SPECT as FDOPA has in PET, and IBZM be compared with raclopride. Concerning the latter two tracers

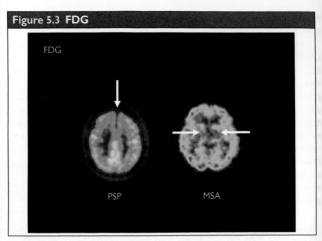

Figure 5.3 FDG

Figure 5.3 Typical examples of cross-sectional brain images of glucose utilization (after application of the [F18] radiolabeled tracer fluoro-deoxy-glucose (FDG) in a patient with PSP (progressive supranuclear palsy) and MSA (multiple system atrophy). Apart from global decreases it can be seen that mediofrontal energy metabolism is decreased in the PSP patient (vertical arrow) and that striatal energy metabolism is decreased in striatum bilaterally (horizontal arrows).

(which are receptor binding substances) in particular, many pharmacological studies have been undertaken. This is a logical consequence of the involved biochemical properties but mainly has significance in the field of research and is not dealt with here. Many remarks made above for PET are also applicable to SPECT. The best-known SPECT tracer for the 'presynaptic' striatal dopaminergic system is FP-CIT radiolabelled with the single photon emitting isotope Iodine-123. FP-CIT binds to the sites at the dopaminergic nerve terminal where synaptically released dopamine is transported back into the nerve terminal. The binding of the tracer to these sites behaves in a dynamic equilibrium fashion but it needs to be emphasized that these transport sites are not receptors. In any event these sites do on the one hand naturally decrease in number when dopaminergic nerve terminals disappear within the context of brain degenerative disorders. On the other hand these sites can also up- or downregulate in numbers due either to disease processes or because of drug interference. Therefore drugs that bind to these transport sites, e.g. the commonly used antidepressants of the class SSRI, can falsely result in a low specific tracer uptake. This will usually affect the whole striatum and not separate regions within. Research projects can make u of these drug-site interactions but in clinical practice it is of im tance to know that the patient has stopped the relevant medication for a sufficient time period.

In practice FP-CIT is used much more often than FDOPA because of the larger availability worldwide of SPECT systems. However, the scan results are comparable from a clinical point of view between the two tracers, although direct comparisons of both tracers in the same patient groups have been made on only a few occasions. The easier availability of FP-CIT SPECT may also be accompanied by disadvantages such as indiscriminate use, without being able to interpret scan results adequately. For instance it is mandatory to have good reference values for each tracer available and this is not pursued everywhere and then the scan results are based solely on visual impressions. This brings to the surface the question of effectivity of sophisticated scanning methods in terms of costs and medical advance. The reader is referred to the published literature.

5.4 Sonography

5.4.1 Introduction

The use of transcranial B-mode ultrasound to assess the echogenicity of brain stem and other structures has been investigated over recent decades. In particular, PD patients will show an increase of the echogenicity of the substantia nigra regions in the brain stem. Hyperechogenicity is concluded if the planimetrically measured area of the echogenic signal within a defined region of the brain is larger in the patient than in the general population or if the visually rated intensity of the ultrasound signal is increased as compared to the surrounding tissue. Thus the method is semiquantitative. However, sophisticated analysis is being developed to ease and standardize the registration. Also, technical developments may improve the method in the future. The method is often referred to as a 'structural' method, but it needs to be remembered that the information is based solely on an ultrasound signal which reflects structure only partially and in the case of, e.g. substantia nigra relates probably to iron content.

To be able to obtain a useful signal technically advanced systems need to be used. Also, an experienced operator is required to perform the measurement adequately. The main disadvantage of the method is the difficulty of obtaining a good temporal acoustic bone window. This means that around 5–10% of Caucasian individuals' midbrain regions cannot be assessed adequately. The basal ganglia regions can not be visualized well in 10–20% of white subjects. In subjects of Asian ethnic origin insufficient bone windows were found in 15–60%. The advantages of the method are non-invasiveness, wide availability, real-time measurement, short investigation times, and independence from subject movements.

5.4.2 Parkinson's disease

Hyperechogenicity of the substantia nigra has been found in up to 90% of patients with PD. In one study a positive predictive value of around 86% had been found. Six of 42 patients who had clinical features of PD had no hyperechogenicity. A hyperechogenic signal of the substantia nigra is usually assumed if the measured area is larger than 0.25 cm^2. About 10% of healthy subjects do, however, show these values. Below 0.20 cm^2 is considered normal, although 10% of the healthy population also has hypoechogenicity. Very elderly healthy subjects show a higher frequency of hyperechogenicity of up to 25%. The definition is dependent on the type of system being used which requires the establishment of own reference values in each laboratory.

The echo signal was not associated with disease severity and did not change with disease progression in a five year follow-up study. This might possibly allow one to detect PD at an early stage of the disease, but monitoring of disease progression cannot be achieved using this method.

Essential tremor patients do not normally show hyperechogenicity of the substantia nigra, but an appreciable subgroup of essential tremor patients will develop PD at a later age and those subjects will possibly be recognized by increased substantia nigra echogenicity.

5.4.3 Other conditions

Depression may be associated with a decreased echogenicity of the midbrain raphe. It has been found that 40–60% of patients with unipolar depression had low echogenicity of the raphe and were responsive to serotonin-reuptake inhibitors. Perhaps there is also a connection with urge incontinence in patients with PD.

In typical cases of multiple system atrophy with parkinsonism (MSA-P) hyperechogenicity of the substantia nigra is seen only rarely, and in patients with progressive supranuclear palsy (PSP) this is found in about a third of the patients. On the other hand, the lentiform nucleus does often show hyperechogenicity. The latter is only seldom seen in PD. Combining the outcome of the echo signal from substantia nigra and lentiform nucleus can therefore differentiate between PD, MSA-P, and PSP: increased signal from substantia nigra and normal signal from lentiform nucleus has a positive predictive value of 0.91 for PD, whereas normal substantia nigra and increased lentiform nucleus signal has a positive predictive value of 0.96 for MSA-P and PSP combined. However, the method cannot distinguish between PD and corticobasal ganglion degeneration (CBGD) since two out of three CBGD patients show an increased substantia nigra signal.

References and further reading

Berg D., Godau J., Walter U. (2008) Transcranial sonography in movement disorders. *Lancet Neurol.* **7**, 1044–55.

Duchesne S., RollandY., Vérin M. (2009) Automated computer differential classification in Parkinsonian Syndromes via pattern analysis on MRI. *Acad. Radiol.* **16**(1), 61–70.

Eckert T. and Eidelberg D. (2005) Neuroimaging and Therapeutics in Movement Disorders. *The Journal of the American Society for Experimental NeuroTherapeutics* **2**, 361–71.

Eshuis S.A., Jager P.L., Maguire R.P., Jonkman S., Dierckx R.A., Leenders K.L. (2009) Direct comparison of FP-CIT SPECT and F-DOPA PET in patients with Parkinson's disease and healthy controls. *Eur. J. Nucl. Med. Mol. Imaging.* **36**(3), 454–62.

Piccini P., Brooks D.J. (2006) New developments of brain imaging for Parkinson's disease and related disorders. *Mov. Disord.* **21**(12), 2035–41.

Scherfler C., Schwarz J., Antonini A., Grosset D., Valldeoriola F., Marek K., Oertel W., Tolosa E., Lees A.J., Poewe W. (2007) Role of DAT-SPECT in the diagnostic work up of parkinsonism. *Mov. Disord.* **22**(9), 1229–38.

Seppi K. (2007) MRI for the differential diagnosis of neurodegenerative parkinsonism in clinical practice. *Parkinsonism Relat. Disord.* **13**(3), S400–5.

Stoessl A.J. (2009) Radionuclide scanning to diagnose Parkinson disease: is it cost-effective? *Nat Clin Pract Neurol.* **5**(1), 10–1.

Chapter 6

The management of early Parkinson's disease

Anthony H.V. Schapira and Anette Schrag

Key points

- Treatment for PD should not be unreasonably delayed, and should be initiated to maintain function and quality of life.
- Drug selection for early PD is determined by individual patient characteristics including severity of symptoms, age, co-morbidity including presence or not of cognitive dysfunction.
- MAOB inhibitors are easy to use and well tolerated, may improve longer term motor outcome, but have a relatively mild symptomatic effect in early PD.
- Dopamine agonists are easy to use (now once a day oral therapies), very effective in improving PD symptoms and delay the onset of motor complications. Side effects e.g. cognitive or behavioural may limit use in a proportion of patients.
- Levodopa is the most effective drug to improve PD symptoms. Its use is limited by the later development of motor complications (wearing-off, dyskinesias).

6.1 Introduction

The diagnosis of Parkinson's disease (PD) rests upon the manifestation of specific motor features, e.g. bradykinesia, rigidity, tremor that are predominantly, although not exclusively, the consequence of dopaminergic cell degeneration in the substantia nigra. It is proposed that by the time clinical diagnosis is possible, pathological changes in the form of Lewy body deposition have already occurred elsewhere in the brain, e.g. olfactory bulb and medulla. Such pathology may underlie some of the clinical pre-motor features of PD, e.g. olfactory ss or rapid eye movement sleep behaviour disorder. Thus it is clear t the pathogenetic processes that lead to nigral cell loss develop considerable time before clinical diagnosis; various parameters st this is at least seven to eight years.

Once the diagnosis of PD is made (see Chapters 3 and 4), the next important decision is when to begin therapy. The patient and their carer require information about the nature of PD, patient support groups, the availability of the different forms of treatment, their benefits and side effects, the prognosis of PD, and general advice about the advantages of exercise.

6.2 **Treatment at diagnosis?**

The traditional view has been that drugs for PD are only of symptomatic benefit and therefore they can be started when the symptoms of PD interfere with social, domestic, or professional life. The patient may be the best judge of this time, although the physician must be alert to inappropriate reluctance to begin medication, and the unnecessary prolongation of disability and impaired quality of life. However, this traditional approach is now challenged and increasingly treatment is offered at diagnosis. The advantages of early treatment include:

1. symptomatic relief
2. potentially improved long term motor outcome.

6.3 **Symptomatic relief**

There is nothing to be gained from withholding treatment from those patients who have significant disability. Likewise, those patients with symptoms that may be mild but which impact significantly upon their social or professional lives will need treatment. The issue for these groups is which drug should be used for initiation (see below).

A more challenging issue is when to begin treatment for those patients with only mild symptoms and no significant functional interference with life. PD patients seek medical attention because of the significance of the symptoms of their disease and some argue that on this basis alone, they should be offered treatment. It is important for the patient to be made aware of the potential improvements that they may derive from treatment. Bradykinesia, rigidity, pain, and sometimes even tremor respond dramatically to dopaminergic drugs. Drug treatment has often been delayed because of concern regarding a decline of medication efficacy over time, or alternatively the development of complications or side effects. The introduction over the past few years of a range of effective and well-tolerated agents renders such concerns less critical. However, the cost of medication, particularly in those health economies where the patient must bear some or all of the expense, can play a role in determining the timing of introduction. In this context it is legitimate for treatment to be delayed at the patient's request, but only to the point at which there is an effect upon social or professional life.

6.4 **Improving long term motor outcome**

Perhaps the most important unmet need in PD is the availability of a drug or intervention to slow or halt progression of the disease and both motor and non-motor symptoms. Although much research effort has gone into developing neuroprotective drugs for PD, none have been able to provide unequivocal evidence of benefit in this regard. Nevertheless, novel concepts of aetiology, pathogenesis, and disease progression have laid the basis for new agents and clinical trial designs to investigate neuroprotection in PD.

The drugs that have received most attention in relation to neuro-protection include the monoamine oxidase (MAO) type B inhibitors and dopamine agonists; although others including co-enzyme Q_{10}, growth factors, anti-apoptotic agents, and glutamate inhibitors have also been the subjects of clinical trials in PD.

6.4.1 **MAO-B inhibitors**

Selegiline (deprenyl) and rasagiline, both MAO-B inhibitors, have demonstrated neuroprotective efficacy in the laboratory and have undergone clinical trials for a disease modifying effect in early PD.

The first of these was the DATATOP study, a prospective double blind, placebo-controlled, trial that investigated the effect of selegiline 5 mg twice daily and/or 2000iu vitamin E as putative neuroprotective therapies. The time until PD patients required levodopa was used as the primary endpoint. No beneficial effect of vitamin E was detected at the dose given. In contrast, selegiline significantly delayed the need for levodopa compared to placebo, an effect consistent with slowing of disease progression. However, selegiline was also found to exert a mild symptomatic effect that confounded interpretation of the study. A long term follow up study of the DATATOP cohort found that selegiline prior to starting levodopa was associated with slower decline, less motor fluctuations and freezing, but more dyskinesias. Whether this was due to selegiline's symptomatic effect or a neuro-protective effect remains unclear. Other studies, on the other hand, did not find a prolonged symptomatic benefit of the combination of levodopa and selegiline compared to levodopa alone with respect to disability or motor fluctuations and dyskinesias. Although one study suggested that selegiline use might be associated with excess mortality, the effect was not seen on longer-term follow-up and a large meta-analysis did not confirm such an effect.

Rasagiline is a more potent MAO-B inhibitor than selegiline. It too has demonstrated protective effects against a wide range of neurotox-ns both in *in vitro* and in *in vivo* studies. Based upon the pre-clinical ta, rasagiline's potential for disease modification was assessed in a el trial design of 'wash-in' or 'randomized start'. The TEMPO study mized patients with early PD to placebo or rasagiline 1 or 2mg and evaluated progression with change from baseline in UPDRS scores over six months. After this time, patients in the placebo group were placed on 2 mg rasagiline and all groups were followed for a further six months. At the end of the study, the change in UPDRS motor score between baseline and final visit was greater in patients who were randomized to the placebo group and received only six months of rasagiline in comparison to those who had received rasagiline for the entire 12 month period. The interpretation of the TEMPO result is complex. The results cannot be explained by a symptomatic effect alone as patients in all groups were receiving the drug at the end of the study. At face value, they represent an early disease modifying effect whereby 12 months of rasagiline had a greater effect than 6.

The results of a large (n>1000) randomized start study (ADAGIO) similar in design to TEMPO have recently been published (Olanow et al. 2009). This study confirmed that patients initiated on 1 mg rasagiline as opposed to placebo for the first nine months maintained improved motor function compared to placebo starters even after all patients had been on the drug for a further nine months.

6.4.2 Dopamine agonists

Dopamine agonists were introduced for their ability to relieve the dopaminergic related motor symptoms of PD. As a drug class, however, they have properties that have potential to provide disease modification and like MAOB inhibitors have demonstrated a variety of protective actions in laboratory studies.

Two studies have sought to determine whether the neuroprotective benefits of dopamine agonists seen in the laboratory can be transferred to patients to modify the course of PD. The CALM-PD study used beta-CIT SPECT to follow the rate of loss of dopamine transporter as a marker of dopaminergic nigrostriatal cell density. Patients with early PD were randomized to pramipexole or levodopa and followed for a total of four years. Levodopa supplementation was allowed in both arms. At two, three and four years there was a significant reduction in the rate of transporter loss in the pramipexole group, averaging out at approximately 40%, consistent with the drug having a relatively protective effect in comparison to levodopa. A similar result was seen in the REAL-PET ropinirole study that used a similar trial design but utilized PET to follow loss of nigrostriatal cell density with fluorodopa. This demonstrated a circa 34% reduction over two years in the ropinirole group compared to those on levodopa. These studies have generated considerable interest and debate. The results are of great interest but, due to uncertainties i the interpretation of PET/SPECT changes in patients on treatme do not prove a neuroprotective effect.

The ELLDOPA trial investigated the possibility that levodopa may be toxic in PD patients. In this study, untreated PD patients were randomized to a total daily dose of 150mg, 300mg or 600mg of levodopa or placebo. Clinical change and Beta-CIT SPECT were used as end-points for integrity of the nigrostriatal system. Levodopa was associated with a significant increase in the rate of decline of the imaging marker over nine months compared to placebo, consistent with a toxic effect. Clinical evaluation, however, showed that those patients on levodopa had better UPDRS scores compared to placebo after two weeks of washout. This would, in contrast, be indicative of a protective effect of levodopa.

6.4.3 Co-enzyme Q10

Coenzyme Q10 has been evaluated in a pilot study of early PD patients to determine whether it might have disease-modifying capabilities. The rationale for the use of coenzyme Q10 in PD was based upon the observation that mitochondrial complex I activity is decreased in the PD substantia nigra. Patients were randomized to either a placebo arm or one of three doses of coenzyme Q10 (300 mg, 600 mg or 1,200 mg) and followed for 16 months. There was a significant benefit for coenzyme Q10 1,200 mg in terms of change from baseline in total UPDRS compared to placebo at 16 months, and a non-significant trend to benefit for lower doses. This interesting and important result is sufficient to support further study of coenzyme Q10, but insufficient at present to advocate that PD patients should use this compound.

6.4.4 Compensatory changes

The clinical onset of PD motor features is directly associated with a series of functional changes in basal ganglia circuits and their target projections. Basal ganglia output becomes abnormal and clinical features appear when dopamine levels fall to <7% in 1-methyl-4-phenyl-1, 2, 3, 6-tetrahydropyridine (MPTP)-treated non-human primates. The corresponding figure in humans is not known, but may be around 20–30%. The estimated asymptomatic latent period of approximately seven to eight years in idiopathic PD indicates the remarkable capacity for the basal ganglia to cope with progressively lower levels of dopamine, the compensatory mechanisms maintaining apparently normal motor function over the intervening years to diagnosis. These compensatory mechanisms include increased striatal dopamine turnover and receptor sensitivity, up-regulation of striatopallidal enkephalin levels, increased subthalamic excitation of the globus pallidus pars externa, and maintenance of cortical motor area activation. These observations, although neither completely defined nor understood, support the notion that declining dopamine levels during the early phase of PD put the basal ganglia level under stress. The onset of clinical symptoms denotes the point of failure to deal adequately with dopamine depletion. It might be that early correction of the basal ganglia functional abnormalities caused by dopaminergic cell loss and dopamine deficiency is a means to support the intrinsic physiological compensatory mechanisms and both limit and delay the circuitry changes that evolve as PD progresses. Review of the outcomes of the DATATOP, ELLDOPA, TEMPO, and ADAGIO studies support such a proposition. In these studies, those patients who received effective symptomatic treatment earlier in the course of their PD fared significantly better clinically than those initiated on placebo even when, as in the case of TEMPO or ADAGIO, they were switched to the active drug after only six or nine months respectively.

Overall, in consideration of when to initiate treatment, the symptomatic benefit of dopaminergic drugs in addition to their potential to improve long term motor outcome, favour their early rather than later introduction. For some patients this could be considered appropriate at diagnosis, for others later initiation might be preferable. Consideration should be given to balancing the benefits outlined above with the potential drawbacks including side effects of medication (see Section 6.5).

6.5 **Which drugs should be used first?**

Drugs available for the symptomatic relief of the motor features of PD include dopaminergic agents, e.g. levodopa, dopamine agonists, MAOB inhibitors, and others such as anti-cholinergics and amantadine. The choice of which of these to use for initial therapy will be determined by a number of factors, most importantly the patient's individual characteristics. The benefits of a drug need to be offset against its short and long-term side effects and complications, and these in turn may vary according to the patient population.

6.5.1 **Levodopa**

This was the first of the dopaminergic drugs and remains the 'gold standard' against which the efficacy of others are judged. Levodopa and other dopaminergic agents improve the quality of life and likely life expectancy of PD patients. It provides rapid and effective relief of bradykinesia, rigidity and associated pain, and improves tremor in many patients. Symptoms such as postural instability, speech disturbance, sialorrhea, etc. may not be improved and represent some of the non-dopaminergic components of PD.

Common early side effects with levodopa are mainly gastrointestinal and comprise nausea, vomiting, and anorexia. These side effects disappear with time, usually over two to three weeks, but may persist in some patients. They can be prevented or treated with domperidone 10–20 mg thrice daily, taken usually for a period of two to four weeks. Constipation, orthostatic hypotension, hallucinations, and daytime sleepiness are less common and are seen more often in the elderly population.

In early disease, levodopa has a long duration response that enables adequate symptomatic control with dosage schedules of three times daily. Disease progression, however, erodes the utility of levodopa as 70% of patients develop motor complications within six years of initiation of the drug. Wearing off effects frequently require modification of dosage and/or dose frequency, or the introduction of additional or alternative therapies.

Another significant long-term complication of levodopa use is the development of dyskinesias which together with 'wearing off', constitute the motor complications caused by levodopa. Dyskinesias develop at a rate of approximately 10% per annum, although this rate is much greater in young onset PD patients, 70% of whom will have dyskinesias within three years of levodopa initiation. The mechanisms by which these motor complications develop are not completely understood but pulsatile stimulation of dopamine receptors by short acting agents including levodopa, and the degree of striatal denervation have been implicated. Dyskinesias may occur at the time of maximal clinical benefit and peak concentration of levodopa (peak dose dyskinesias) or appear at the onset and wearing off of the levodopa effect (diphasic dyskinesias). Motor complications can be an important source of disability for some patients who cycle between 'on' periods which are complicated by dyskinesias and 'off' periods in which they suffer severe parkinsonism.

6.5.2 **Dopamine agonists**

Several dopamine agonists are available for use in PD and fall broadly into two groups: ergot and non-ergot. Ergot agonists include bromocriptine, cabergoline, lisuride, and pergolide, non-ergot agonists include apomorphine, piribedil, ropinirole and pramipexole. These drugs have been the subjects of extensive evaluation in clinical trials. Bromocriptine, cabergoline, pergolide, pramipexole and ropinirole have all been studied for monotherapy use in early PD as well as for adjunctive treatment in more advanced PD. Although the effect on motor improvement is less than on levodopa, they have all demonstrated a significant beneficial effect on motor function and activities of daily living. Their side effect profile is similar to levodopa in terms of inducing dopaminergic related symptoms such as nausea, vomiting, and postural hypotension, but are associated with a higher rate of peripheral oedema, somnolence (relevant especially for drivers), and hallucinations, particularly in the elderly.

The use of dopamine agonists is rarely associated with the development of pleural, pericardial, or peritoneal fibrosis. Recent studies have also demonstrated an increased risk of the ergolinic dopamine agonists pergolide and cabergoline with fibrotic cardiac valvular disease, in a pattern similar to that seen with other agents that also stimulate the 5HT-2 receptor, including methysergide and fenfluramine. The effect may be dose-related. Patients receiving these drugs should be actively monitored with echocardiography for the development of these complications. Whether switching to a non-ergot dopamine agonist prevents further progression and whether this effect is reversible after discontinuation is currently unclear. In addition, the question whether this complication also occurs with other ergot agonists without 5HT(2B) activity requires further study. Dopamine agonists have also been associated with behavioural changes such as impulse control disorders, e.g. hypersexuality, gambling, or shopping. Younger patients appear to be more at risk and need to warned about these potential side effects, which are dose-dependent and reversible with medication withdrawal.

Dopamine agonist monotherapy can effectively control dopaminergic symptoms for a period of time. Long-term follow-up indicates that approximately 85%, 68%, 55%, 43%, and 34% of PD patients initiated on pramipexole or ropinirole are still controlled on monotherapy at one, two, three, four, and five years respectively. However, this is dependent upon the agonist being used at an appropriate dose. Several trials have now confirmed that bromocriptine, cabergoline, pergolide, pramipexole, and ropinirole are associated with a significantly reduced risk for the development of motor complications in comparison to levodopa. Nevertheless, patients will require levodopa supplementation at some point during their disease, and long-term data suggest that the difference in motor complications between those initially started on levodopa or on bromocriptine is not maintained at 14 years.

In conclusion, dopamine agonists provide effective control of PD related motor symptoms, delay the onset of motor complications, delay the introduction of levodopa, and enable a lower dose of levodopa to be used.

6.5.3 MAO-B inhibitors

Selegiline has been extensively studied for symptomatic benefit in early and advanced PD. Meta-analysis of 13 randomized trials showed that this drug has a mild anti-parkinsonian effect. Selegiline delays the need for additional dopaminergic therapy by nine to 12 months in early PD and once introduced, levodopa dose is lower in those patients remaining on selegiline. Rasagiline improves the motor features of early PD and this effect lasts about six months, at which point patients have returned to their baseline score. Thus MAO-B inhibitors offer a viable option for initial therapy in early PD. The symptomatic benefit is significant but relatively modest, although it is greater in those patients with more motor disability. The ability to delay levodopa introduction is important in terms of retarding the development of motor complications. The disease modifying effect, although unproven, offers an additional potential advantage.

6.5.4 **Other drugs**

Anti-cholinergics have been used to treat the symptoms of PD since before the introduction of levodopa. Relatively little data are available on potency and tolerance. Clinical trials have shown a modest benefit for anti-cholinergics in improving parkinsonism, but this was at the expense of impaired cognitive function, particularly in the elderly.

Amantadine produces mild improvement in PD symptoms, with benefits usually lasting 6 to 9 months. It is generally considered unsuitable for monotherapy in PD and is mostly used as an adjunct. Improvements in bradykinesia and rigidity are generally of the same order of magnitude as anti-cholinergics, but their combination is additive. Amantadine use is also limited by its potential to induce cognitive defects. However, amantadine has been reported to improve treatment-related dyskinesias and is therefore also used as an adjunct in advanced disease with dyskinesias (see Chapter 7).

6.5.5 **A practical approach to the initiation of drug treatment in PD**

The patient's age and the presence of any cognitive impairment or significant co-morbidity that is likely to influence life expectancy or medication tolerance are important early considerations in deciding initial therapy for PD. Most PD patients come to diagnosis early in their seventh decade; patients recruited to the dopamine agonist monotherapy studies were mean age 61–62 years. For these and especially for the younger onset patients, symptomatic control can be an important issue as many are still at work. They are also at greater risk of the development of motor complications with levodopa, and any possibility of disease modification will hold special attraction. Their disease is likely to run for 15 to 20 years or more and there is the opportunity early on to lay the foundations for an effective, safe and well tolerated long-term treatment strategy.

Approaches to PD management in various stages are presented below. These represent the views of the authors.

(i) Early PD with onset below age 70 years.

    (a) In those patients whose PD symptoms are only mild but who desire some improvement in function, it is suggested that these patients are offered a MAO-B inhibitor or a dopamine agonist as first line therapy.

    (b) If PD symptoms are more significant and/or symptomatic improvement is required, patients with no evidence of cognitive impairment should be initiated on a dopamine agonist or levodopa following information on the potential advantages and disadvantages of each.

(ii) Early PD with onset over age 70 years.

Generally, patients over age 70 years are increasingly less tolerant of dopamine agonists, although a significant proportion of patients this age and older can still benefit from agonist use with an acceptable side effect profile. Cognitive impairment can be considered a relative contraindication to dopamine agonist use as these drugs carry a higher risk of confusion and hallucinations. PD patients over age 70 have a relatively lower rate of onset of dyskinesias than younger patients, but these can still develop at about 5–10% per annum.

(a) Patients aged 70 to 75 years should be carefully evaluated and if otherwise in good health, and without cognitive dysfunction, should be offered a dopamine agonist or levodopa following information on the advantages and disadvantages of each, and followed to ensure they are able to tolerate the medication well.

(b) Patients with cognitive deficits or comorbities that are likely to be exacerbated by dopamine agonists who require symptomatic control of their PD should be initiated on levodopa.

(c) Patients over the age of 75 years should be offered levodopa as first line treatment for their PD symptoms.

The principle underlying these recommendations is to provide effective symptom control appropriate to the patients' needs and to minimize the short and long term side effects of therapy.

6.6 **Second line therapy**

Those patients initiated on a MAO-B inhibitor will at some point require additional therapy in order to control their motor symptoms. The addition of a dopamine agonist is usually the most appropriate second line treatment for these patients, so long as they remain free of cognitive disturbance and do not require or choose levodopa. However, studies addressing the degree of benefit provided by a dopamine agonist and rasagiline together have not yet been performed.

Patients initiated on a dopamine agonist should have their dose titrated to maximal effect over time in order to maintain their motor control. As indicated above, these patients will at some point require supplementary medication. A choice can then be made between introducing a MAO-B inhibitor or levodopa. Although the combination of a dopamine agonist and rasagiline has not been studied, rasagiline is well tolerated and has been shown to improve control in early patients and those stable on levodopa, improving 'on' time and reducing 'off' time to a degree equivalent with entacapone. The addition of rasagiline might enable a further delay in the introduction of levodopa. Inevitably, however, levodopa will be required as disease progression results in accumulating motor deficit.

When levodopa is added, the MAO-B inhibitor or dopamine agonist should be continued unchanged, unless side effects necessitate dose reduction or withdrawal.

The concomitant administration of a catechol-O-methyl transferase (COMT) inhibitor to levodopa, either separately as entacapone or tolcapone, or in combination as Stalevo® (levodopa and a dopadecarboxylase inhibitor with entacapone) offers an alternative approach to prolongation of the action of levodopa. At the time of writing, data on the effect of this combination therapy (which is effective in advanced disease) in early disease are not available.

In conclusion, the introduction of second line therapy in PD may be necessary in order to maintain control of motor features and improved quality of life. The choice of drug used at this stage depends upon the characteristics of the patient and the medication used to date, as well as the nature of their motor decline and the presence or absence of motor fluctuations. The following is recommended by the authors as a practical guide for clinicians.

(a) Those patients initiated on a MAO-B inhibitor should be offered a dopamine agonist or levodopa when additional therapy becomes necessary, unless they are cognitively impaired, over 75 years of age, or choose or require levodopa, in which case they should be given levodopa as the second drug.

(b) Those PD patients initiated on a dopamine agonist who reach the stage of requiring additional therapy may derive some additional benefit from rasagiline.

(c) Levodopa will be necessary for those on a dopamine agonist with or without rasagiline who require additional symptom control. If possible we suggest that this is introduced as a three or four times a day regimen. There are theoretical reasons and some experimental data to support the introduction of levodopa in combination with entacapone, although this position cannot formally be advocated pending the results of clinical trials currently underway.

(d) The greatest choice is for those patients already on levodopa who require additional control or who are experiencing wearing off. If started on levodopa because of cognitive impairment, comorbidity, age over 75 years disease severity, or choice, the simplest approach is to increase the daily dose of levodopa with a frequency of administration four to six times daily. However, this may be impractical for some patients in this group and for them the use of entacapone or Stalevo offers the benefit of extended and enhanced symptom control with the potential for a simplified dose regimen. Other patients who do not have relevant comorbidities or cognitive impairment may benefit from introduction of dopamine agonist treatment at this point, thereby improving control and motor fluctuations, maintaining a lower dose of levodopa and delaying dyskinesias. Additionally, the use of rasagiline is another optional and will provide additional benefit to those on levodopa with or without motor fluctuations. The course of action selected will depend much on the characteristics of the patient and the severity and stage of the PD.

6.7 **Conclusions**

This chapter has sought to provide a practical guide to management options for the various stages of PD. It has already been emphasized by us and the other contributors to this book that treatment needs to conform to the individual needs of the patient. In addition, the patient must be involved as much as is both possible and reasonable in the decision-making process, particularly in the timing of the initiation of drug treatment and the nature of first-line therapy. The physician and patient have several options available, each with their own advantages and disadvantages, this chapter should hopefully enable the selection process to be as informed as possible.

References and further reading

Goetz C.G., Poewe W., Rascol O., Sampaio C. (2005) Evidence-based medical review update: pharmacological and surgical treatments of Parkinson's disease: 2001 to 2004. *Mov Disord.* **20**(5), 523–39.

Horstink M., Tolosa E., Bonuccelli U., Deuschl G., Friedman A., Kanovsky P., Larsen J.P., Lees A., Oertel W., Poewe W., Rascol O., Sampaio C.; European Federation of Neurological Societies; Movement Disorder Society-European Section. (2006) Review of the therapeutic management of Parkinson's disease. Report of a joint task force of the European Federation of Neurological Societies and the Movement Disorder Society-European Section. Part I: early (uncomplicated) Parkinson's disease. *Eur J. Neurol.* **13**, 1170–85.

Olanow C.W., Rascol O., Hauser R., et al. (2009). A double-blind, delayed-start trial of rasagiline in Parkinson's disease. *N Engl J Med.* **361**(13), 1268–78.

Pahwa R., Factor S.A., Lyons K.E., et al. (2006) Quality Standards Subcommittee of the American Academy of Neurology. Practice Parameter: treatment of Parkinson disease with motor fluctuations and dyskinesia (an evidence-based review): report of the Quality Standar

Subcommittee of the American Academy of Neurology. *Neurology*, **66**(7), 983–95.

Schapira A.H. (2007) Treatment options in the modern management of Parkinson disease. *Arch Neurol.*, **64**(8), 1083–8.

Schapira A.H., Obeso J. (2006) Timing of treatment initiation in Parkinson's disease: A need for reappraisal? *Ann Neurol.* **59**, 559–62.

Schapira A.H., Olanow C.W. (2004) Neuroprotection in Parkinson disease: mysteries, myths, and misconceptions. *JAMA*, **291**(3), 358–64.

Stowe R.L., Ives N.J., Clarke C., van Hilten J., Ferreira J., Hawker R.J., Shah L., Wheatley K., Gray R. (2008) Dopamine agonist therapy in early Parkinson's disease. *Cochrane Database Syst Rev.*, **16**, CD006564.

Chapter 7

Medical management of motor complications

D.A. Gallagher and Anthony H.V. Schapira

> ## Key points
>
> - The development of levodopa-related motor complications is related to the dose and duration of levodopa use, the age of patient and severity of disease.
> - The initial use of dopamine agonists delays the onset of motor complications.
> - MAOB inhibitors, COMT inhibitors and dopamine agonists are all effective in treating wearing off. Modifications of levodopa use: increased dose or frequency may also be appropriate in some patients.
> - Amantadine is useful to reduce dyskinesias. Apomorphine or duodopa can be considered for selected patients. Surgery is beneficial for appropriate individuals.

7.1 Definitions and prevalence of motor complications

The motor phenotype of Parkinson's disease (PD) is characterized by tremor, rigidity, bradykinesia, and gait disturbance and results from dopamine depletion in the substantia nigra pars compacta. In the early phase following diagnosis, levodopa administration results in a consistent and effective improvement in motor symptoms, despite the relatively short half-life of this drug (60–90 minutes). Effective symptom control can often be achieved at a dosing frequency that would be insufficient to achieve sustained motor benefit in later disease, and patients are often able to omit medication doses with little discernible deterioration in motor function. This phenomenon is termed the long duration response (LDR). As disease progresses, motor fluctuations can emerge which encompass periods where dopaminergic medication results in good symptomatic benefit ('on'

63

state) and periods where the effect of dopaminergic medication diminishes with the re-emergence of debilitating motor symptoms ('off' state). The 'off' state is often initially manifested as the 'wearing off' phenomenon, where the apparent duration of action of dopaminergic medication decreases, termed the short duration response (SDR). An increased frequency dosing schedule is required and any delay or omission of a drug dose is likely to result in development of the 'off' state. The 'off' state can, however, occur in other circumstances. 'Dose failure' is the term applied to the failure to achieve any symptomatic benefit ('on' response) from a dose of levodopa. Contributory factors include autonomic dysfunction inherent to PD (abnormal gastrointestinal peristaltic activity affecting drug absorption) and competitive intestinal membrane transport with other dietary amino acids. Motor fluctuations can also occur rapidly (within a few seconds, termed 'sudden onset off') or in an unpredictable manner (not clearly related to the timing of dopaminergic medication, termed 'unpredictable off'), immediately following taking medication 'beginning of dose effect', or in a diurnal pattern (including increasing predisposition to 'off' state as day progresses or morning time amelioration of symptoms, termed 'sleep benefit').

Dyskinesias represent involuntary movements (choreiform, ballistic, or dystonic) which can occur at peak plasma concentrations of dopaminergic medications ('peak dose dyskinesia') but can also occur during the entire 'on' period ('square wave dyskinesia'), or at the beginning of dose (when plasma concentrations are increasing) and at the end of dose (decreasing plasma concentrations), termed 'diphasic dyskinesia'. During the 'wearing off' period or in the 'off' state, patients may describe painful sensations related to dystonic posturing of the limbs and this is particularly prevalent in the early morning ('early morning dystonia').

Predicting the latency to development and the type of motor complications that will occur in any given individual with PD is difficult and is dependent on a number of variables, including disease-related factors (young-onset versus older onset PD, mono-allelic genetic forms versus idiopathic PD), severity of motor symptoms, treatment onset (immediate versus delayed) and dopaminergic drug type (levodopa, dopamine agonist, etc). It is estimated from analysis of the published literature that approximately 50% of patients will experience motor complications within four to six years. However, evidence from clinical drug trials of monotherapy in early PD suggest that these complications can emerge soon after initiation of therapy, particularly with high dose ($\geq$ 600mg/day) of levodopa. Overall it is estimated that there is a cumulative 10% risk per year of developing motor complications in PD.

7.2 Pathogenesis of motor complications

7.2.1 Pharmacodynamics and pharmacokinetics

The pathogenesis of motor complications in Parkinson's disease is not fully understood but is likely to involve a complex interaction of pre-synaptic and post-synaptic effects. A non-linear pattern of substantia nigra dopamine loss has been demonstrated in autopsy studies and in longitudinal studies using functional imaging ([^{18}F]fluorodopa Positron Emission Tomography, PET) or clinimetric rating scales (Unified Parkinson's Disease Rating Scale, UPDRS) as surrogate markers for nigral cell loss. It is estimated that a least 50% of dopaminergic neurones will have been lost in the substantia nigra before the onset of significantly discernible motor symptoms and data from these studies have been extrapolated to suggest a pre-motor phase in PD of approximately six to eight years. Redundancy or neuroplasticity in dopaminergic neurotransmission have been invoked to explain this phenomenon, the latter being the most likely explanation.

Homeostatic modifications that have been demonstrated include development of new synaptic terminals, increased turnover of endogenous dopamine and neuronal firing, regulation of dopamine transporter (DAT) and dopaminergic autoreceptors, upregulated expression of post-synaptic dopamine receptors, increased expression of nerve trophic factors, and alteration of glial interactions (Linazasoro, 2007). Interactions with other neurotransmitter systems, including glutamate-amino butyric acid (GABA), adenosine, acetylcholine, serotonin, and opioid receptors have also been implicated. Experimental and clinical studies have suggested a role for these non-dopaminergic neurotransmitter systems in modifying the pharmacodynamic response of the dopamine receptor complex to endogenous dopamine or dopaminergic pharmacotherapies. For example, in primates with 1-methyl-4-phenyl-1, 2, 3, 6-tetrahydropyridine (MPTP) induced parkinsonism, serotoninergic agents (including the 5-HT$_{1A}$ agonist sarizotan and the 5-HT$_{2A}$ and 5-HT$_{2C}$ antagonists quetiapine and clozapine) can dramatically reduce levodopa-induced dyskinesias (LID). In clinical studies clozapine (5-HT$_{2A}$ and 5-HT$_{2C}$ antagonist) and mirtazapine (5-HT$_{1A}$ agonist and 5-HT$_{2A}$ antagonist properties) have shown some benefit in reducing LID. N-methyl-D-aspartate (NMDA) receptor antagonists such as amantadine have shown some benefit in reducing LID. Pre-clinical primate models of PD and studies in humans suggest therapeutic potential for adenosine A$_2$ receptor antagonists in improving motor complications. In addition, there is likely modification of downstream G-protein coupled second messenger systems. These homeostatic mechanisms and pharmacodynamic alterations are proposed to underpin the maintenance of normal motor function despite nigrostriatal degeneration in the pre-motor phase of PD (allowing a pre-symptomatic phase of up to

6-8 years or more) and continued response to exogenous levodopa during the 'honeymoon period' (consistent and effective response to dopaminergic medication) despite progressive neurodegeneration. However this creates a non-physiological neurobiological substrate in which the phenomena of *sensitization* and *tolerance* can occur, ultimately leading to a predisposition to motor fluctuations and dyskinesias.

Others have proposed that pre-synaptic effects predominate. A mathematical model based on in vivo dynamic PET studies (de la Fuente-Fernandez, 2007) has been proposed to explain motor complications in PD. In the context of neurodegeneration and dopaminergic cell loss, exogenous dopamine (metabolized from levodopa) has progressively fewer nerve terminals for uptake and recycling into synaptic vesicles. Thus the observed association between disease progression and severity of motor complications in PD. Individual differences in dopamine release rate (encompassing vesicle release rate and vesicular quantal dopamine content) have been used to explain predisposition to develop motor complications. For example, the predilection of patients with young onset PD for motor complications may be related to higher dopamine release rate compared to older patients and therefore greater rate of synaptic dopamine loss.

It is likely that both pre-synaptic and post-synaptic alterations and pharmacokinetic and pharmodynamic effects are important in the development of motor complications, and will provide important pharmacological targets for future drug therapies in PD.

7.2.2 **Continuous dopaminergic stimulation**

It is postulated that motor fluctuations and dyskinesias can be delayed or diminished by dopaminergic stimulation in a more physiological manner, termed continuous dopaminergic stimulation (CDS). This has led to the development of longer acting preparations of currently available pharmacotherapies (a controlled release preparation of the dopamine agonist pramipexole is currently undergoing clinical evaluation and controlled-release ropinirole has recently become available) and novel methods of administration including continuous intra-duodenal levodopa infusions and the trans-dermal dopamine agonist patch rotigotine.

A recent review (Nutt, 2007) has examined the assumptions inherent to the CDS hypothesis and its *in vivo* applicability to PD. Namely, (1) CDS is physiological and therefore drugs should be developed to have pharmocokinetics to achieve constant plasma levels, (2) motor complications result from sensitization caused by pulsatile dopaminergic stimulation (a phenomenon exemplified by drugs with short plasma half lives, such as levodopa), and (3) continuous administration of dopaminergic agents will not lead to clinically problematic tolerance.

Each of these assumptions has been considered. Firstly, phasic increases in striatal dopmine concentration in response to physical activity have been demonstrated in microelectrode studies in rats and by functional imaging (increased displacement of the radiolabelled dopamine receptor antagonist raclopride in PET studies and iodobenzamide in single photon emission computer tomography, SPECT study). However, whilst dopaminergic stimulation is unlikely to be truly constant, CDS more closely approximates to the physiological state than the several fold variations in dopamine concentrations in response to exogenous dopamine, particularly in the denervated state.

Secondly, the pulsatile nature of levodopa pharmacokinetics is proposed as a cause of *sensitization* which would explain levodopa-induced dyskinesias and the short-duration response (decreased latency and increased magnitude of peak motor response) demonstrated in PD. However, motor fluctuations are more easily explained in terms of levodopa *tolerance* and rightward shift of the levodopa dose-response curve with disease progression which has been demonstrated in human subjects.

Thirdly, development of tolerance in response to CDS is a potential concern. Reduced response to levodopa or apomorphine boluses following continuous levodopa or apomorphine infusions respectively and decremental responses to repeated apomorphine doses has been demonstrated. Therefore, in clinical practice continuous subcutaneous apomorphine infusions are given with nocturnal breaks to prevent tolerance and allow re-sensitization.

7.3 Drug and surgical treatments

7.3.1 Delaying onset of motor fluctuations and dyskinesias

Although there is an emerging consensus that treatment for PD should be started earlier rather than later, there is debate regarding which dopaminergic agent should be used as initial monotherapy. The decision depends on individual patient circumstances, particularly age, cognition, degree of disability, predisposition to drug-related side effects (including nausea, autonomic dysfunction or neuropsychiatric sequelae) and potential for development of long-term motor complications (fluctuations and dyskinesias). Options for initial monotherapy in PD include the monoamine oxidase B (MAO-B) inhibitors selegiline and rasagiline, synthetic dopamine agonists or levodopa in combination with a decarboxylase inhibitor.

The newer non-ergot derived dopamine agonists have generally superseded older ergot alternatives due to concern about cardiopulmonary fibrotic complications, with the later. Randomized controlled trials comparing these newer dopamine agonist treatments (pramipexole, CALM-PD study and ropinirole, REAL-PET study) with levodopa as an initial treatment for motor symptoms in PD, have demonstrated greater clinical efficacy for levodopa (demonstrated by improvement on UPDRS) but reduced frequency and delayed emergence of motor complications with dopamine agonists. There is evidence that this risk is related to cumulative levodopa dose and total levodopa-equivalent dose. The relatively short half-life of levodopa compared to dopamine agonists, and therefore more pulsatile stimulation of dopamine receptors, has been given as an explanation for this observation and is often given in support for the CDS theory. However, this pharmacokinetic approach is likely to be too simplistic an explanation, given the different post-synaptic receptor profiles of these drugs.

Nonetheless, these studies demonstrate that individual drugs and drug classes used as monotherapy in early PD have differing capacity to induce long-term motor complications and that this is an important consideration when initiating therapy in PD.

Traditionally pharmacological treatment in PD has been delayed for as long as possible to avoid development of motor complications. This convention has recently been challenged by the emergence of newer dopaminergic drug therapies and studies with novel designs that suggest that sustained motor benefit can be achieved with early drug treatment. For example, a double blind randomized controlled trial of the MAO-B inhibitor rasagiline using a 'delayed start' protocol (TEMPO study) and a double blind trial comparing levodopa and placebo, followed by a period of washout (ELLDOPA study) have suggested early treatment may confer long term benefit on motor function. Two studies comparing levodopa with the newer non-ergot derived dopamine agonists ropinirole and pramipexole, with functional imaging endpoints as a marker of dopaminergic neurone loss (ropinirole versus levodopa, using [18F]fluorodopa PET, REAL-PET study and pramipexole versus levodopa, using [123I]-βCIT SPECT) suggest sustained benefit with initial dopamine agonist treatment compared to levodopa.

The clinical application of these studies is limited by the complex interpretational considerations of functional imaging in PD (PET and SPECT) and limitations in the use of clinimetric scales as markers of dopaminergic function. Nonetheless, current clinical evidence would imply that early monotherapy with the MAO-B inhibitor rasagiline, the dopamine agonists ropinirole and pramipexole, and even levodopa, may confer long term motor advantages compared to placebo. This creates a dilemma, given the association of early dopaminergic drug treatment with increased risk of developing motor fluctuations and dyskinesias.

It is currently unclear whether administration of dopaminergic medication in a manner more consistent with the CDS hypothesis in early PD results in delayed onset of motor complications. Entacapone increases the elimination half-life of levodopa and is proposed to produce a more physiological pharmacokinetic plasma profile. However, this increase in levodopa half life is probably insufficient to reduce the risk of dyskinesias through CDS unless the preparation was to be given at a frequency that would likely be impractical for PD patients.

7.3.2 Evidence for medical treatment of motor fluctuations

An evidence based review by the Quality Standards Subcommittee of the American Academy of Neurology (AAN) (Pahwa et al., 2006) has examined the medical and surgical treatments for levodopa-induced motor complications in PD. A comprehensive literature search was performed and all clinical trials examined were stratified according to strict criteria. The highest level of evidence (class I) was defined as prospective randomized studies with blinded and clearly defined primary outcome measure assessments, clearly defined inclusion and exclusion criteria, sufficiently few drop-outs to minimize bias and equivalent baseline characteristics between treatment groups.

The catechol-O-methyltransferase (COMT) inhibitor entacapone and MAO-B inhibitor rasagiline have received the highest level of recommendation (class A, established to be effective, requiring at least two class I studies). For entacapone in this systematic review, two class I studies demonstrated significant improvement in 'on' time compared to placebo, but in one there was a significant increase in dyskinesia. In addition a Cochrane Database Systematic Review of controlled trials of entacapone (eight trials, N=1560) demonstrated a weighted mean difference of 'on' time of 1.5 hours (95% confidence interval [CI] 1.2 to 1.7). However, this meta-analysis also revealed an increased risk of dyskinesia although this could be managed by reduced concomitant dopaminergic therapy (odds ratio [OR] 3.1, 95% CI 2.6 to 3.7). Other complications more frequently encountered in the entacapone group were nausea, vomiting, diarrhoea, constipation, hallucinations and dizziness.

Two class I studies of the MAO-B inhibitor rasagiline (PRESTO study and LARGO study) have compared rasagiline to placebo as an adjunct in levodopa treated patients with motor fluctuations and have demonstrated significantly reduced 'off' time, but in one study increased risk of dyskinesia. Rasagiline is a newer MAO-B inhibitor which is considered to have a more favourable side-effect profile than selegiline. However, reported side effects in these studies included nausea, anorexia, dizziness, orthostatic hypotension, hallucinations and sleep disturbances.

The dopamine agonists pramipexole, ropinirole, and pergolide and the COMT inhibitor tolcapone received the second level of recommendation (class B, probably effective, requiring at least one class I study or two consistent class II studies). Pramipexole demonstrated efficacy in reducing 'off' time in one class I and one class II study, but there was increased dyskinesia in both. Ropinirole showed effectiveness in decreasing 'off' time in two class II studies, one of which demonstrated significant increase in dyskinesia however the second study did not comment on this complication. Pergolide demonstrated effectiveness in one class I study. The older ergot-derived dopamine agonists have been generally superseded by newer non-ergot derivatives (ropinirole, pramipexole, and trans-dermal rotigotine) due to concerns for cardiopulmonary fibrotic complications associated with the former. Side-effects of dopamine agonists include nausea, somnolence (including reports of irresistible sudden onset 'sleep attacks'), orthostatic dizziness, visual hallucinations, and impulse control disorders (hypersexuality, pathological gambling, excessive shopping, and eating).

Two class II studies have shown improvement in 'off' time with tolcapone. Tolcapone has a similar side-effect profile to entacapone but has additionally been associated with derangement of liver function, and in rare cases fatal hepatotoxicity. For this reason its licence was revoked in several countries but it is now licenced for use in patients whose motor fluctuations have not responded to other adjuvant therapies provided frequent monitoring of liver function is made.

Subcutaneous apomorphine, oral cabergoline (an ergot-derived dopamine agonists) and selegiline (MAO-B inhibitor) received class C recommendation suggesting possible but unproven clinical effectiveness. Bromocriptine and levodopa controlled release preparations were felt to have no influence on motor complications.

Since the completion of this systematic review, several new preparations of previously available dopaminergic drugs (for example intra-duodenal levodopa and controlled release formulation of ropinirole) and novel dopaminergic molecules (trans-dermal dopamine agonist rotigotine) with pharmacokinetic profiles more consistent with CDS have become available. In a large (506 participants) well designed double-blind placebo-controlled trial comparing rotigotine with pramipexole and placebo (CLEOPATRA-PD study, Poewe et al., 2007) rotigotine and pramipexole demonstrated similar efficacy in reducing 'off' time (2.5 hours and 2.8 hours respectively) in PD patients experiencing motor fluctuations. The ropinirole 24 hour controlled release preparation has demonstrated efficacy in reducing 'off' time in a large (393 subjects) double blind placebo-controlled trial in patients experiencing motor fluctuations (Pahwa, 2007).

In several small open label studies, intra-jejunal levodopa (Solvay Duodopa®) has demonstrated reduced 'off' time, improved dyskinesia, and improved overall quality of life. In a single small double-blind study (ten participants) of jejunal levodopa, seven patients had improvement in motor fluctuations. Administration of jejunal levodopa has specific additional considerations, including requirement for an invasive procedure to insert a percutaneous gastrostomy/jejunostomy. Therefore, levodopa infusions are generally reserved for advanced cases of motor fluctuations in whom several other pharmacotherapies have been tried and failed.

7.3.3 Evidence for medical treatment of dyskinesias

A small (24 participants) and short (three weeks) double blind placebo-controlled crossover trial of amantadine as treatment for LID demonstrated 24% reduction in total dyskinesia score (P=0.004). Therefore amantadine is possibly effective in reducing LID in PD (AAN recommendation level C) but further large well designed clinical trials will be needed to confirm its efficacy.

7.3.4 Surgical treatments for motor complications

The evidence based review by the Quality Standards Subcommittee of the AAN also examined the effect of surgical interventions including deep brain stimulation (DBS) of the subthalamic nucleus (STN), globus pallidus interna (GPi) and ventral intermediate nucleus of the thalamus (VIM). Due to the invasive nature of this treatment, absence of control population (sham surgery) and small number of participants in most studies, the highest evidence level found was level III (DBS of STN, four class III studies and DBS of GPi, one class III study). The DBS studies have consistently demonstrated marked improvements in 'off' time and reduction in dyskinesias. However, because of the lack of high evidence level studies, the AAN gives class C recommendation (possibly effective) for DBS of the STN. In addition, given the small number of trials for DBS of the GPi and VIM, the AAN felt that there was insufficient evidence to make any recommendations for clinical effectiveness.

DBS involves invasive surgical intervention and there are additional complications related to this. DBS can result in surgical and perioperative complications, including haemorrhage, infection, anaesthesia associated complications, thromboembolic disease, and permanent neurological deficits. Mechanical complications including lead displacement, malfunction or fracture should also be considered.

7.4 Conclusion

Motor complications are common in PD, their prevalence related to dopaminergic drug use and disease duration. Various mechanisms have been proposed, both pharmacokinetic and pharmacodynamic and involving pre-synaptic and post-synaptic alterations. The most appropriate time to initiate treatment in PD is unclear but a potential long-term benefit from early treatment counterbalanced by the predilection to develop long-term motor complications must be considered. Different dopaminergic medications (in particular dopamine agonists versus levodopa) result in different predispositions to develop motor complications. It is uncertain whether drugs with pharmacokinetics that produce CDS can protect from or delay the development of motor complications. Systematic analyses of published clinical trials suggest that the MAO-B inhibitor rasagiline and the COMT inhibitor entacapone have the highest evidence for reduction of motor complications (class A recommendation). The COMT inhibitor tolcapone and the dopamine agonists are also likely to be effective (class B recommendation). There is evidence from a small double blind trial that amantadine may be effective in reducing dyskinesias.

References and further reading

de la Fuente-Fernández R. (2007) Presynaptic mechanisms of motor complications in Parkinson disease. *Arch Neurol.* **64**(1), 141–3.

Fox S.H., Lang A.E. (2008) Levodopa-related motor complications—phenomenology. *Mov Disord.* **23**(3), S509–S14.

Linazasoro G. (2007) Pathophysiology of motor complications in Parkinson disease: postsynaptic mechanisms are crucial. *Arch Neurol.* **64**(1), 137–40.

Nutt J.G. (2007) Continuous dopaminergic stimulation: Is it the answer to the motor complications of Levodopa? *Mov Disord.* **22**(1), 1–9.

Pahwa R., Factor S.A., Lyons K.E., Ondo W.G., Gronseth G., Bronte-Stewart H., Hallett M., Miyasaki J., Stevens J., Weiner W.J. (2006) Quality Standards Subcommittee of the American Academy of Neurology. Practice Parameter: treatment of Parkinson disease with motor fluctuations and dyskinesia (an evidence-based review): report of the Quality Standards Subcommittee of the American Academy of Neurology. *Neurology* **66**(7), 983–95.

Schapira A.H. (2007) Treatment options in the modern management of Parkinson disease. *Arch Neurol.* **64**(8), 1083–8.

Schapira A.H., Bezard E., Brotchie J., Calon F., Collingridge G.L., Ferger B., Hengerer B., Hirsch E., Jenner P., Le Novère N., Obeso J.A., Schwarzschild M.A., Spampinato U., Davidai G. (2006) Novel pharmacological targets for the treatment of Parkinson's disease. *Nat Rev Drug Discov.* **5**(10), 845–54.

Schapira A.H., Obeso J. (2006) Timing of treatment initiation in Parkinson's disease: a need for reappraisal? *Ann Neurol.* **59**(3), 559–62.

Chapter 8

Management of non-motor symptoms of Parkinson's disease

Shyamal H. Meta and Kapil D. Sethi

Key points

- Patients with Parkinson's disease (PD) may suffer from non-motor symptoms at all stages of the disease. At times, patients find the non-motor symptoms more distressing than the motor symptoms of PD
- Olfactory dysfunction, constipation and impaired visuospatial discrimination may occur even before the appearance of motor symptoms
- The non-motor symptoms of PD can be attributed to the involvement of multiple neurotransmitter systems including the dopaminergic system in the degenerative process. In general, these symptoms are unresponsive to dopaminergic therapy and require different treatment strategies
- Failure to recognize impulse control disorders in patients on dopaminergic therapy (especially dopamine agonists) may result in significant adverse consequences.

8.1 Introduction

Parkinson's disease (PD) is the second most common chronically progressive neurodegenerative disease, behind Alzheimer's disease (AD). Since James Parkinson's first description of the disease in 'An Essay on the Shaking Palsy', cardinal motor features such as tremor, bradykinesia and rigidity have been intensely studied and have led to effective treatment of these symptoms. However, even in his first monograph in 1817, Dr. Parkinson recognized several non-motor features such as sleep disturbance, bowel and bladder problems, and delirium in his patients with the disease. In spite of this, the non-motor symptoms (NMS) of PD had largely been on the 'back burner' until recently. Multiple studies have shown the widespread prevalence of NMS in PD patients and many, if not all patients suffer from NMS. (Gulati *et al.* 2004, Hely *et al.* 2005, Poewe 2007). Contrary to earlier belief, NMS are not only a feature of advanced disease but are also commonly seen in early stages and in many cases may predate the development of motor symptoms and the clinical diagnosis of PD.

Rightfully so, increasing attention to NMS from neurologists and movement disorder specialists has led to the development of quantifiable scales to assess the burden of NMS in PD. Results from such questionnaire type studies have shown that NMS cause significant impairment of quality of life, sometimes more so than the motor symptoms of the disease (Gulati *et al.* 2004, Hely *et al.* 2005). Common NMS seen in PD (albeit not a comprehensive list) are outlined in Box 8.1. As far as understanding the etiology of NMS in PD is concerned, it is now widely recognized that the pathology in PD extends beyond the nigrostriatal dopaminergic system. Recent work by Braak and colleagues suggests that degeneration in non-dopaminergic regions (particularly the dorsal motor nucleus and olfactory regions) precedes the development of dopaminergic pathology, and this in turn may account for why non-motor features such as sleep disturbances, impaired olfaction and constipation precede the onset of the classic motor features of PD. As multiple neurotransmitter systems are perturbed in PD, many of the NMS remain levodopa unresponsive and their treatment remains a challenge.

8.2 Management of non-motor symptoms of Parkinson's disease

The first step in management is vigilance in recognition of NMS by the treating clinician as these can be frequently overlooked. A prospective study involving 101 PD patients showed that during routine office visits, neurologists failed to identify the presence of depression, anxiety, and fatigue more than half the time and failed to recognize sleep disturbance in 40% of patients (Shulman *et al.* 2002). Hence, assessing the NMS either subjectively or quantitatively with questionnaires such as NMSQuest, etc. is a crucial first step in the management of these symptoms.

The next important step is to discern the cause of the particular symptom. Some of the NMS may be a consequence of advancing PD whereas other symptoms like impulse control disorders (ICD, particularly in patients on dopamine agonists) may be related to side effects of PD medications and some (like orthostatic hypotension) may be a combination of both. In such cases, management strategies may vary from modifying the dopaminergic medication as well as the addition of a non-dopaminergic medication.

Box 8.1 Common non-motor manifestations of Parkinson disease

Autonomic symptoms
Orthostatic hypotension
Urogenital dysfunction
- Bladder problems: urgency, nocturia, frequency
- Sexual dysfunction: erectile dysfunction

Sweating
Gastrointestinal symptoms
- Constipation
- Hypersalivation
- Dysphagia
- Nausea
- Fecal incontinence

Neuropsychiatric symptoms
Mood disorders
- Depression
- Anxiety
- Apathy
- Anhedonia

Mild cognitive impairment and dementia
Behavioral disorders
- Impulse control disorders
- Punding

Psychosis:
- Hallucinations
- Delusions
- Illusions

Sleep disorders
Insomnia
Frequent night time awakenings
Excessive daytime sleepiness
REM behavior sleep disorder
Restless legs syndrome

Sensory disturbances
Pain
Olfactory disturbances

Miscellaneous
Fatigue
Diplopia
Weight loss/gain

We lack evidence based on clinical studies in a homogenous PD population, therefore the treatment is largely empiric based on small studies and expert opinion.

Autonomic dysfunction

...nomic dysfunction is a common feature of PD affecting several ...dy systems such as the cardiovascular, urogenital and gastrointes-...nal systems. The estimated prevalence of autonomic dysfunction in PD ranges from 14–80% and autonomic symptoms are more common in PD patients as compared to controls across all stages of the disease. The cause of autonomic symptoms in PD is related to pathology in both the peripheral and central nervous system, as well as dopaminergic therapy. Some of the more common autonomic symptoms are outlined below:

8.2.1.1 *Orthostatic hypotension*

The prevalence of symptomatic orthostatic hypotension (OH) in PD patients varies from 30 to 58%. Although more common in advanced PD, it can also be seen in early stages. However, marked dysautonomia early in the course of the disease should raise a strong suspicion of the diagnosis of multiple system atrophy (MSA). Symptoms include postural lightheadedness with fainting or falls and occasionally jerking of the body. OH is related to postganglionic sympathetic and cardiac baroreflex dysfunction. Also, dopaminergic therapy or treatment with other vasodilators such as tamsulosin (for bladder problems) or doxazosin (for hypertension) may cause OH.

There is a lack of controlled studies in the treatment of OH in a homogenous PD population. Available studies have involved mixed populations of patients with neurogenic hypotension. Current management strategies involve using a combination of physical measures and pharmacological agents for the treatment of OH. A detailed diary of at-home measurement of supine and upright blood pressure and pulse can be extremely helpful in the evaluation and treatment of patients. Physical measures include the use of elastic stockings, head-up tilt while lying down and getting up gradually especially in the postprandial period. In addition, the patients should be advised to increase fluid and salt intake. Drugs that worsen OH such as tamsulosin and doxazosin should be stopped and antihypertensive treatment in patients who were previously hypertensive should be re-evaluated. Two groups of drugs with different mechanism are utilized to treat OH. These include mineralocorticoids such as fludrocortisone 0.1–0.3 mg/day to increase sodium and fluid reabsorption and sympathomimetic agents (alpha adrenergic stimulants) such as midodrine 2.5–10 mg/day or etilefrine 15–25 mg/day. Supine hypertension is a potential side-effect of all of the above mentioned drugs, especially the alpha adrenergic stimulants. Therefore, patients should be advised not to lie down flat for two to three hours after the administration of such agents. Phase III, randomized, controlled trials using novel agents such as atomoxetine and L-threo-3,4-dihydroxyphenylserine (L-threo-DOPS) for treatment of neurogenic

OH are currently underway. These trials are recruiting patients with several disorders causing OH including PD.

8.2.1.2 *Urogenital dysfunction*

A wide variety of urological symptoms may occur in PD. These include a wide range from urinary urgency and frequency, incomplete bladder emptying to incontinence. PD patients also suffer from sexual dysfunction including erectile dysfunction and ejaculatory failure in men and decreased libido and inadequate lubrication in women. It may be difficult to differentiate PD related urological problems from age related dysfunction due to associated disorders such as prostate enlargement, etc. Once urogenital problems have been discovered, one must work in consultation with a urologist and proper diagnostic testing to potentially identify reversible/treatable causes should be undertaken The treating physician must also pay attention to other medications such as antidepressants (SSRI) or antihypertensive/cardiac medications (beta-blockers), all of which can cause sexual dysfunction.

Usually, urogenital dysfunction is a late feature of PD as opposed to MSA, where it is often seen within the first year of symptom onset. The most common abnormality of micturition in PD is due to detrusor hyperrelexia (stimulation of detrusor muscle contractions at low urine volumes otherwise not seen normally).

Anticholinergics (oxybutynin 5–15 mg/day, tolterodine 2–4 mg/day or trospium chloride 20–40 mg/day) are the most commonly used agents to treat detrusor hyperreflexia in PD. Tolterodine and trospium are preferred to oxybutynin in advanced PD due to a decreased propensity to worsen cognitive dysfunction in this patient population. This is attributed to the fact that trospium chloride does not cross the blood-brain barrier and tolterodine is comparatively less lipophilic. A newer anticholinergic (muscarinic antagonist) solifenacin succinate, used as once daily dosing (5–10 mg/day), has been shown to be effective in treating symptoms of overactive bladder and a large scale clinical trial in PD patients in being planned. However, like the other anticholinergic agents, this drug can cause side effects such as dry mouth, confusion, and constipation.

Studies have also shown improvement of bladder capacity and decrease in the symptoms of overactive bladder in PD patients following subthalamic nucleus (STN) stimulation.

As mentioned earlier, sexual dysfunction is frequently seen in patients with PD. However, it remains one of the more poorly investigated areas of PD. Sexual dysfunction in PD is multi-factorial and probably related to a combination of aging, PD pathology, interpersonal relationships, comorbid depression and medications (such as antidepressants). Bronner *et al.* investigated sexual function in patients with PD: women reported difficulties with arousal, with reaching an orgasm, with low sexual desire, and with sexual dissatisfaction; men reported erectile dysfunction, sexual dissatisfaction, premature ejaculation, and difficulties in reaching an orgasm (Meco et al. 2008). Using a Quality of Sexual Life Questionnaire (QoSL-Q), Moore et al. found that the quality of sexual life was significantly reduced in all PD patients and correlated with disease progression and aging (Moore et al. 2002).

As far as treatment of sexual dysfunction is concerned, working in consort with a urologist and gynecologist to identify and treat reversible causes is important. A randomized, placebo-controlled trial found sildenafil (50 mg) to be effective in improving erectile dysfunction in PD patients. Other phosphodiesterase inhibitors, such as vardenafil (10 mg) and tadalafil (20 mg) have also been used in clinical practice to treat erectile dysfunction in patients with PD. As an alternative to phosphodiesterase inhibitors, apomorphine (a dopamine agonist) has also been used. Both the injectable and the sublingual formulation (3 mg/dose), have shown benefit in treatment of sexual dysfunction in addition, to improving the motor symptoms of PD. However, phosphodiesterase inhibitors and apomorphine may result in or worsen orthostatic hypotension. Treatment options for sexual dysfunction in women are limited and confined to sexual education and behavior therapy, use of estrogen for dyspareunia due vuvlovaginal atrophy and more recently testosterone gel for hypoactive sexual desire disorder. Phosphodiesterase inhibitors have shown to be of limited benefit in women in small studies.

8.2.1.3 *Constipation*

Constipation is a very common complaint in PD and related to the poor GI motility. Defining constipation as less than three bowel movements per week, a survey from 2002 found ~20% of PD patients suffer from constipation. In the Honolulu Heart study, men who reported having less than one bowel movement daily had a risk of developing PD 2.7 times higher than that of men with daily bowel movements, and four times higher than that of men who had two or more bowel movements a day suggesting that constipation is an early manifestation of PD pathology or that constipation somehow predisposed individuals to developed PD in the future (Pfeiffer 2003). Since constipation does not respond to dopaminergic therapy, non-dopaminergic mechanisms may be implicated. Anticholinergics such as trihexyphenidyl and benztropine used in PD can also worsen constipation and may need to be stopped. Along similar lines, newer drugs such as mosapride and tegaserod (5-HT$_4$ agonists) can stimulate release of acetylcholine and enhance GI motility. These drugs are currently under investigation (although tegaserod has recently been withdrawn from the market). Practical lifestyle modifications such as adequate intake of liquids and dietary fibre may ameliorate some symptoms o constipation. In a double blind clinical trial using psyllium (a fib supplement), stool frequency improved significantly in PD patients. Addition of laxatives (polyethylene glycol, lactulose or sorbitol) and stool softeners such as docusate may also be beneficial. Recently, lubiprostone (24 mcg/day), a locally acting chloride channel activator in the intestine, has been approved for treatment of chronic idiopathic constipation. Although, there is no data in PD patients, future studies with this drug are warranted.

8.2.1.4 *Mood disorders*

The prevalence of major depression in PD ranges from 4–70% in different studies with a mean of ~40%. PD patients with depression have less guilt, fewer self-destructive thoughts and rarely commit suicides as compared to patients with primary major depression. On the other hand, anhedonia, anxiety, and panic attacks are encountered more frequently. Based on the Braak hypothesis, multiple neurotransmitter deficiencies related to PD pathology play a role in causing depressive symptoms. Studies suggest that depression may precede the motor symptoms of Parkinson's disease in up to 30% of the patients.

In the management of depression in PD, a combination of psychotherapy with pharmacotherapy is always a prudent approach. Counseling and adequate discussion at the time of diagnosis is important to allay anxiety and concerns associated with getting diagnosed with PD. The two broad categories of pharmacotherapy involve dopaminergic medication used in PD and/or traditional antidepressant drugs in general use for depression. Mood swings, anxiety, and feeling of panic can all be associated with 'wearing off' state in PD and needs to be investigated. In such a situation, optimizing dopaminergic therapy is the mainstay of treatment. Other PD medications such as selegiline, a MAO-B inhibitor have been shown to exert a potent antidepressant effect. Dopamine agonists such as ropinirole and pramipexole may also have antidepressant properties based on various animal studies, due to their action on the D2/D3 receptors. A randomized, parallel group trial comparing pramipexole to sertraline in PD patients on stable levodopa dose and without any motor fluctuations, showed that both drugs significantly reduced depressive symptoms, although pramipexole was more effective in terms of number of recovered patients. A large randomized, double-blinded, placebo controlled trial of pramipexole in PD depression was recently completed, and preliminary results show that the drug is effective in treating PD depression. (NCT00297778).

Currently, traditional agents such as tricyclic antidepressants (TCA) and selective serotonin reuptake inhibitors (SSRI) are the most common drugs used to treat depression in PD. A placebo-controlled, randomized study using nortriptyline was done ~20 years ago. It owed a significant improvement in depression over placebo. Subsequent randomized controlled trials with SSRI such as citalopram vs. placebo and sertraline vs. placebo, failed to show a significant difference between the drug and placebo groups. Other uncontrolled trials with SSRI such as paroxetine (20 mg/day) showed a statistically significant improvement in depression based on rating scales as compared to placebo.

Newer agents such as reboxetine and venlafaxine have been used in practice to treat PD associated depression, however, clinical studies with these agents are largely lacking as with other newer antidepressants such as mirtazapine.

Although electroconvulsive therapy (ECT) has been around for a long time for the treatment of refractory depression, data in PD depression is scarce. However, anecdotal reports suggest that it is efficacious and safe.

In general, some of the principles of treatment of PD-associated depression from our practice are as follows: actively inquiring about the symptoms of depression at each office visit as patients may not recognize symptoms or know that they have underlying depression, focus on optimal control of motor symptoms of PD with adequate dopaminergic therapy to see if it improves depressive symptoms, in the absence of significant randomized, controlled data, add-on treatment with SSRI/TCAs or newer agents (based on side-effect profile and individual tolerance of each drug). Referral to a psychiatrist should be sought if these measures fail to control depression.

8.2.1.5 Dementia and psychosis

Cognitive impairment in PD ranges from subtle deficits early on such as bradyphrenia, word finding difficulty and problems with planning and goal-directed behaviors to development of dementia with worsening disability. Parkinson's disease-dementia (PDD) has a reported prevalence of 20–44% with a wide variability. Prevalence as high as ~90% can be found in PD patients in nursing homes. Development of dementia in PD is associated with more rapid progression of disability, increased risk of nursing home placement and increased mortality. A recent concept in the field of PDD is the introduction of mild cognitive impairment (MCI) where the subjects have milder forms of cognitive dysfunction not severe enough to meet diagnostic criteria for dementia, i.e. MCI is a pre-clinical state of dementia. A significant amount of research to better define and assess MCI is currently being done.

Cholinesterase inhibitors are the mainstay of drug treatment for PDD. All drugs of this class are probably effective but only the use of rivastigmine is supported by a large scale, randomized, controlled clinical trial in PDD. Daily dose of ~9mg showed significant improvement of cognitive functioning as assessed by rating scales and care-give interviews. Smaller trials and open label studies using other choli-neasterase inhibitors such as donepezil (10 mg/day), galantamine (8 mg/day) and tacrine have suggested efficacy in PDD. Although, the studies have shown a modest improvement at best, in a group as a whole, individual patients may show significant benefit. Phase III/IV studies using a NMDA receptor antagonist, memantine (20 mg/day) and with safinamide (with cognition as a secondary outcome measure) in PDD are currently underway.

Psychosis affects ~1/3 patients with PD and is commonly associated with cognitive decline. Elderly PD patients can also acutely develop hallucinations due to intercurrent medical illnesses such as dehydration or infections, or as a side effect of dopaminergic or non-dopaminergic drugs such as pain medications, anticholinergic agents, benzodiazepines, etc. One should also re-assess the anti-Parkinsonian drugs as they could also contribute to the psychosis. Drugs should be stopped in the order as shown in Box 9.2. Visual hallucinations seen in advanced PD represent well formed and complex images and situations. These may be stable and non-distressing in some patients and may not require treatment under such circumstances. However, in others, they may be frightening, indistinguishable from reality and accompanied by paranoid or persecutory delusions. The presence of visual hallucinations early in the disease (within first year of symptom onset) should raise suspicion for a diagnosis of Dementia with Lewy bodies (DLB). Treatment options of psychotic symptoms in PD include using atypical antipsychotic agents such as quetiapine or cloza-pine based on The Movement Disorders Task Force consensus statement made after reviewing the evidence for various antipsychotics. Older typical antipsychotics such as haloperidol, etc are not recommended due to their extrapyramidal side effects from the strong binding to the D2 receptors. Newer atypical agents such as risperi-done and olanzapine should be avoided due to worsening of PD motor symptoms. Both, clozapine and quetiapine should be started at low doses and slowly titrated to achieve the desired clinical effect. Typical doses are significantly lower than the ones used in schizophrenia. Monitoring for side effects is crucial with these agents as sedation can occur with both and clozapine can cause a fatal agranulocytosis (requiring blood count monitoring) and postural hypotension. Also, neuroleptic malignant syndrome can occur and sudden stopping of these drugs should be avoided.

Another agent, pimavanserin (5-HT$_{2A}$ inverse agonist) is in a Phase III clinical study for improvement of psychosis in PD patients. The phase II study showed promising results with no worsening of PD motor symptoms with its use.

> ## Box 8.2 PD medications worsening psychosis
>
> - Careful review of the PD medications is essential in patients with PD psychosis.
> - Assess risk-benefit ratio of the drug, i.e. extent of resolution of psychosis vs. worsening symptoms of PD from stopping the drug.
> - PD drugs should be stopped in the following order:
>   - Anti-cholinergics
>   - Selegiline
>   - Amantadine
>   - Dopamine agonists
>   - COMT inhibitors
>   - Reduce levodopa dose as last resort (after trying addition of atypical antipsychotics such as clozapine or quetiapine).

8.2.1.6 *Sleep disorders*

Sleep disturbances are unrecognized in over 40% of PD patients. While the exact prevalence of sleep disturbances in patients with PD is not known, sleep complaints have been reported in as many as 60–90% of PD patients. Some PD-specific sleep problems range from excessive daytime sleepiness from dopaminergic therapy to nocturnal immobility, tremor, dyskinesia, periodic and aperiodic limb movements, and RLS. Nocturia can also cause sleep disruption. Selegiline may have an alerting effect and could cause difficulty initiating sleep. Other non-motor symptoms such as depression and psychosis can also interfere with nighttime sleep. The treatment of sleep dysfunction in PD begins with awareness on part of the treating physician. A detailed history regarding the nature of sleep problems should be obtained from the patient along with the care giver (as sometimes the patient maybe unaware of the problems). Further management of the problem rests on determining the proximate cause of sleep disruption (as outlined in Figure 8.1), i.e. night-time akinesia – treat with addition of nighttime dose of dopaminergic therapy or consider a long acting dopamine agonist like rotigotine or long acting ropinirole, REM behaviour disorder – clonazepam at bedtime, psychosis and depression – treat with appropriate medication, excessive daytime sleepiness – decrease dopaminergic dose or addition of stimulants such as modafinil or amphetamines in the morning.

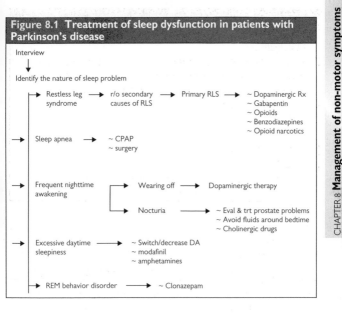

Figure 8.1 Treatment of sleep dysfunction in patients with Parkinson's disease

Interview
↓
Identify the nature of sleep problem

→ Restless leg syndrome → r/o secondary causes of RLS → Primary RLS → ~ Dopaminergic Rx
~ Gabapentin
~ Opioids
~ Benzodiazepines
~ Opioid narcotics

→ Sleep apnea → ~ CPAP
~ surgery

→ Frequent nighttime awakening → Wearing off → Dopaminergic therapy
→ Nocturia → ~ Eval & trt prostate problems
~ Avoid fluids around bedtime
~ Cholinergic drugs

→ Excessive daytime sleepiness → ~ Switch/decrease DA
~ modafinil
~ amphetamines

→ REM behavior disorder → ~ Clonazepam

8.2.1.7 *Behavioral problems: Impulse control disorders and punding*

Impulse control disorders (ICD) such as compulsive eating, pathological gambling and hypersexuality as well as punding (aimless, repetitive activity or manipulations along with a peculiar fascination with certain objects) are increasingly seen in patients with PD on dopaminergic therapy – especially with DA. Lifetime prevalence of ICD is ~14% in PD patients on dopaminergic therapy; whereas punding is much less common (~1.4% in one study). These compulsive behaviors and punding can be a significant source of distress to the patient and his family.

Management of these dopamine related behaviours (DRB) begins with educating the patient and the family about these behaviours. If possible, dose of the dopaminergic medications – especially the DA, should be reduced. While no particular dopaminergic therapy is more prone to cause punding; DA are much more likely to instigate ICD as compared to levodopa. Also, self-administration of 'rescue' or 'as needed' doses of medications by such a patient should be discouraged, to prevent hedonistic homeostatic dysregulation syndrome. Decreasing the dose of dopaminergic medication may worsen PD symptoms. Future dose increases should be judiciously done. Another therapeutic option is to transition the patient to deep brain stimulation (DBS) as treatment of DRB with out compromising motor function.

Antipsychotics and psychotherapy have been studied as adjunctive measures for the treatment of DRB without promising results.

8.2.1.8 *Pain*

Sensory complaints such as pain are a common feature of PD. Pain may more often be related to motor fluctuations such as wearing off or early morning dystonia as opposed to rare neuritic syndromes such as burning mouth or genital pain syndromes. All of the above mentioned pain complaints respond to modifications in their PD drug regimen as opposed to being treated with conventional analgesics. Painful focal dystonia may be treated with injections of botulinum toxin. From a practical standpoint, it is important to identify the most proximate cause of new onset pain such as in the hip, back and other joints as patients with PD fall frequently and may need orthopedic consultation. Rarely, a deep visceral pain associated with retroperitoneal fibrosis due to the use of DA may also be seen which may need surgical intervention.

References and further reading

Chaudhuri K.R., Martinez-Martin P. (2008) Quantitation of non-motor symptoms in Parkinson's disease. *Eur J Neurol.* **15**(2), 2–7.

Comella C.L. (2008).. Sleep disorders in Parkinson's disease. *Curr Treat Options Neurol.*, **10**, 215–21.

Emre M. (2007) Treatment of dementia associated with Parkinson's disease. *Parkinsonism Relat Disord.* **13**(3), S457–S61.

Ferrara J.M. and Stacy M. (2008) Impulse-control disorders in Parkinson's disease. *CNS Spectr.*, **13**, 690–8.

Fox S., Brotchie J.M., Lang A.E. (2008) Non-dopaminergic treatments in development for Parkinson's disease. *Lancet Neurol.*, **7**, 927–38.

Gulati A., Forbes A., Stegie F. et al. (2004) A clinical observational study of the pattern and occurrence non-motor symptoms in Parkinson's disease ranging from early to advanced disease. *Mov Disord.*, **19**(9), S406.

Hely M.A., Morris J.G., Reid W.G., Trafficante R. (2005) Sydney Multicenter Study of Parkinson's disease: non-L-dopa-responsive problems dominate at 15 years. *Mov Disord.* **20**, 190–9.

Kaufmann H. and Goldstein D.S. (2007) Autonomic dysfunction in Parkinson's disease. *Handb Clin Neurol.* **83**, 343–63.

Meco G., Rubino A., Caravona N., Valente M. (2008) Sexual dysfunction in Parkinson's disease. *Parkinsonism Relat Disord.* **14**, 451–6.

Moore O., Gurevich T., Korczyn A.D., Anca M., Shabtai H., Giladi N. (2002) Quality of sexual life in Parkinson's disease. *Parkinsonism Relat Disord.* **8**, 243–6.

Pfeiffer R.F. (2003) Gastrointestinal dysfunction in Parkinson's disease. *Lancet Neurol.* **2**, 107–16.

Poewe W., Seppi K. (2008) Managing the non-motor symptoms of Parkinson's disease. In: Hallett M, Poewe W, eds. *Therapeutics of Parkinson's Disease and Other Movement Disorders.* Wiley-Blackwell. pp. 91–120.

Pramipexole Versus Placebo in Parkinson's Disease (PD) Patients With Depressive Symptoms. http://clinicaltrials.gov/ct2/show/NCT00297778 (accessed on December 11, 2008).

Sethi KD (2008) Levodopa unresponsive symptoms in Parkinson's disease. *Mov Disord.* **23**(3), S521–S33.

Shulman L.M., Taback R.L., Rabinstein A.A., Weiner W.J. (2002) Nonrecognition of depression and other non-motor symptoms in Parkinson's disease. *Parkinsonism Relat Disord.* **8**, 193–7.

Weintraub D., Morales K.H., Moberg P.J. et al. (2005) Antidepressant studies in Parkinson's disease: a review and meta-analysis. *Mov Disord.* **20**, 1161–9.

Zahodne L.B., Fernandez H.H. (2008) Pathophysiology and treatment of psychosis in Parkinson's disease: a review. *Drugs Aging.* **25**, 665–82.

Zesiewicz T.A. Solifenacin Succinate (VESIcare) for the Treatment of Urinary Incontinence in Parkinson's Disease. http://clinicaltrials.gov/ct2/show/NCT00584090 (accessed on December 10, 2008).

Chapter 9

Surgery in Parkinson's disease

Irene Martinez-Torres and Patricia Limousin

Key points

- Surgical treatment for Parkinson's disease is currently dominated by deep brain stimulation (DBS)
- The subthalamic nucleus (STN) has become the target most commonly used in DBS as it improves a wide range of symptoms
- Thalamic or pallidal stimulation still have their places and should not be ignored
- Ablative procedures are considered for selected patients, when DBS is contraindicated or not available
- Neuroprotective and restorative approaches, such as cell transplantation or gene therapy are still in development and might in the future replace DBS.

Neurosurgical treatment for Parkinson's disease (PD) has been carried out for more than a century. The current surgical approach is dominated by deep brain stimulation (DBS); nevertheless ablative procedures are performed for selected patients and in countries where DBS technology is not available. Dopaminergic cell transplantation results have to date been disappointing. Stem cells and gene therapy are still in an early stage of development.

9.1 Deep brain stimulation

DBS is currently the surgical procedure most commonly used for PD. It offers significant benefits in carefully selected patients. DBS involves implanting electrodes in a specific area of the brain that are connected to an implantable pulse generator (IPG) located in the subclavicular area (Figure 9.1).

There are three well established targets: subthalamic nucleus (STN), globus pallidus internum (GPi) and ventro-intermediate nucleus (Vim) of the thalamus (Figure 9.2).

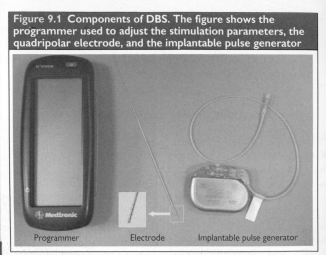

Figure 9.1 Components of DBS. The figure shows the programmer used to adjust the stimulation parameters, the quadripolar electrode, and the implantable pulse generator

Programmer   Electrode   Implantable pulse generator

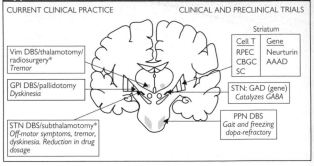

Figure 9.2 Brain targets for the different surgical approaches for Parkinson's disease

CURRENT CLINICAL PRACTICE   CLINICAL AND PRECLINICAL TRIALS

Vim DBS/thalamotomy/radiosurgery*
Tremor

GPI DBS/pallidotomy
Dyskinesia

STN DBS/subthalamotomy*
Off-motor symptoms, tremor, dyskinesia. Reduction in drug dosage

Striatum

Cell T	Gene
RPEC	Neurturin
CBGC	AAAD
SC	

STN: GAD (gene)
Catalyzes GABA

PPN DBS
Gait and freezing dopa-refractory

9.1.1 **Patient selection**

9.1.1.1 *Who can be considered for DBS?*

The first step in the selection of the optimal patient is to establish the diagnosis of idiopathic PD. Patients with atypical parkinsonism need to be excluded as they do not respond to DBS.

- Duration of the disease: a minimum of five years is suggested, mainly to exclude atypical parkinsonism. Surgery could be considered earlier depending on the age and the impact of the symptoms.
- PD severity: motor fluctuations, dyskinesia and/or tremor that are not sufficiently controlled by medication and which produce a negative impact on the quality of life.

- Levodopa-responsiveness: as a general rule, only symptoms that respond to levodopa will respond to DBS. An exception is tremor, which can need excessively high doses of medication and yet responds well to STN or Vim DBS. Other causes of tremor have to be excluded.
- Age: there is no strict cut-off age. Age-related comorbidities are more important than age *per se*. However caution should be exercised with patients over 70 years old, in particular for STN DBS as risks are usually higher for this target.

9.1.1.2 *Contraindications for surgery*

General contraindications for surgery:

- Severe comorbidities, in particular cardiovascular problems
- Severe psychiatric problems: severe depression, suicide attempts, psychosis. These problems are at risk of deteriorating after DBS, especially with STN DBS and should be considered carefully
- Marked cognitive decline
- Neurosurgical contraindications: severe brain atrophy, extensive white matter lesions or lesions in the basal ganglia could increase the risk of intracranial haemorrhage and stroke
- Immunosuppression: risk of hardware infection.

Other considerations: oral anticoagulation has to be stopped when possible or replaced by heparin. Antiaggregant or nonsteroidal anti-inflammatory treatment should be stopped 14 days before and after surgery.

9.1.1.3 *Preoperative evaluation*

- Dopa-challenge. Evaluation of the symptoms off and on-medication using the motor Unified PD rating scale.
- Brain MRI
- Neuropsychometry
- Others when concerns (psychiatric, cardiologist...)

9.1.1.4 *How to predict the response to DBS?*

Patient symptoms have to be assessed extensively. The main disabling symptom needs to be identified and its possible response to DBS determined.

Levodopa responsiveness is the best predictor of a positive response to DBS.

Symptoms that do not respond to levodopa will not respond to DBS and are even at risk of deteriorating.

Gait and balance difficulties, and freezing need to be assessed care-fully. They can worsen after surgery when non dopa-responsive.

Speech response to DBS can be variable. Swallowing and speech can deteriorate if preoperative difficulties exit.

It is important that patients and their families understand the risks and benefits as well as the limitations of DBS. Their expectations have to be realistic and the patient needs to be able to participate in the routine programming of the stimulation.

9.1.1.5 *Selection of the appropriate target: benefits and risks (Table 9.1)*

STN is the preferred target as it improves a wider range of symptoms (off-motor symptoms that respond to levodopa). It allows a reduction in dopaminergic medication and therefore improves also dyskinesia in the long-term.

GPi DBS has less marked impact on off-motor symptoms than STN but has a direct antidyskinetic effect, facilitating the management of drug therapy afterwards.

Vim stimulation is mainly used, usually as unilateral procedure, in tremor-dominant elderly patients who are not disabled by other symptoms. In younger patients with tremor, STN is prefered as other symptoms will appear with the progression of the disease.

STN DBS entails greater risk for cognitive and psychiatric side effects.

Patients considered borderline for STN DBS because of age, psychiatric problems or cognitive dysfunction might still be suitable for GPi and Vim DBS.

9.1.2 **Surgical procedure**

Different methodologies are used depending on the centres. Stereotactic brain MRI is generally performed to calculate targets coordinates. STN and GPi are visible on MRI and target coordinates can be calculated directly. Vim is not visible and requires indirect targeting using atlas coordinates. Presently, quadripolar electrodes are available. Most surgical teams implant the electrodes under local anaesthesia for the STN and Vim, to allow intraoperative stimulation and assessment of side effects, and microrecording if desired. In these cases antiparkinsonian medication is withdrawn the night before. General anaesthesia is generally used for GPi DBS because its acute effect on symptoms is less clear. Once the electrodes have been implanted a new brain imaging (CT or MRI) can be used to verify the position of the electrodes and to rule out surgical complications. The IPG is implanted under general anaesthesia the same day or a few days later. Prophylactic systemic antibiotics are used at the time of the surgery.

The main risks of surgery for all targets are: intracranial haemorrhage (1–4%), infection (1–15%) and rarely seizures. In the early postoperative period transient confusion and psychiatric problems are frequent, especially with STN DBS.

Table 9.1 Criteria for the selection of the target in DBS			
	STN	**GPI**	**VIM**
Indications	Medically intractable MF, Dysk or tremor. Major disability from off-symptoms	Medically intractable MF, Dysk. Major disability from Dysk. When STN is a concern because of age, psychiatric history of cognition	Medically intractable tremor. No major disability from other parkinsonian symptoms. Patients at risk for STN
Effect on:			
Rigidity	+++	+	No effect
	+++	+	No effect
Bradykinesia	+++	+	+++
Tremor	+++*	No effect	No effect
Gait	++†	+++	No effect
Dyskinesias	+++	Variable‡	No effect
↓Drug dosage			
Concerns/ side effects	Balance and gait problems non-dopa responsive. Speech, dysphagia. Psychiatric cognition	Dysarthria, dysphagia. Psychiatric, cognition (less frequent than with STN)	Dysarthria, dysphagia. Ataxia (especially if bilateral). Other symptoms, more disabling than tremor will appear. Risk of tolerance and rebound if 24h stimulation

9.1.3 Postoperative management

A spontaneous improvement in symptoms can be noted before starting the stimulation due to a lesion-like effect produced by the implantation of the electrode. However this effect wears off after a few weeks. Once the patient has recovered from surgery the adjustment of the stimulation parameters can be started.

9.1.3.1 Programming the stimulation

The adjustment of the stimulation parameters are done using an external programmer that connects with the IPG telemetrically (Figure 9.1).

9.1.3.1.1 Stimulation parameters

The stimulation parameters that can be programmed are: amplitude, pulse width, frequency and selection of the electrode's contact

They are similar for the three targets: frequency has to be higher than 100 Hz, and 130 Hz is the most often used; amplitude varies between 2–4 volts; and pulse width is usually set at 60 μs, and tends to be higher for GPi.

Monopolar stimulation (one or more contacts of the electrode as cathode and IPG case as anode) is considered the most effective option.

Bipolar stimulation (one or more contact as cathode and one contact as anode) may be preferred if a narrower current is needed to reduce side effects.

9.1.3.1.2 *First screening session*

Each contact of the electrode is tested for its efficacy on rigidity, bradykinesia, tremor, and gait and for side effects in the off-medication condition.

The amplitude is progressively increased and pulse width and frequency are kept at 60 μs and 130 Hz.

The most effective contact (best clinical effect at lowest amplitude and highest threshold for side effects) is selected.

9.1.3.1.3 *Adjustment of medication and stimulation after the first screening*

STN DBS: amplitude has to be progressively increased along with reduction of dopaminergic medication; otherwise there is a risk of inducing dyskinesia or neuropsychiatric side effects. It is important not to reduce medication too fast or excessively, as this can lead to apathy or depression. Optimal adjustment of stimulation and medication are reached after three to six months.

GPi and Vim DBS: the amplitude can be set faster as no adjustment of medication is usually required.

After each adjustment session the patient has to be reassessed on-medication, especially for the STN and GPi. This will enable to assess the effect of dopaminergic medication and readjust the stimulation in case of excessive dyskinesia.

For Vim DBS some tolerance to the effect of the stimulation overtime has been observed. To prevent this problem patients are advised to switch off the stimulation at night or when it is not needed. A stimulation holiday can also help.

9.1.3.1.4 *Side effects*

Some are related to amplitude of the current and are therefore adjustable.

They are more frequent with STN DBS, especially for cognition and psychiatric problems

Dysarthria has been seen with the three targets and is often related to high amplitudes.

Weight gain and eyelid-opening apraxia are common after STN or GPi DBS.

Neuropsychiatric problems are mainly seen with STN DBS and range from depression and apathy to mania. They can be stimulation-related.

Cognitive decline has been seen after STN DBS (in particular verbal fluency) and GPi DBS especially when older age at baseline.

9.1.4 **Long term follow-up**

Regular follow-up visits are needed to allow adjustment of medication and stimulation and also to monitor malfunctioning, and battery depletion. Visits are more frequent during the first six months.

The existing batteries have to be replaced every four to seven years. The next generation of batteries are likely to last longer and some models will be rechargeable.

Deterioration of symptoms, especially axial symptoms and cognition, has been seen in most of the studies for the three targets, and are likely to be compatible with disease's progression (Table 9.2).

9.1.4.1 *Long-term complications*

Sudden loss of benefit on symptoms can occur with hardware-related complications. These include: lead fracture, lead migration, and battery depletion or battery failure and are estimated at 4.3% per electrode.

Skin erosion, infection of the device related to sepsis may occur at any time.

9.1.4.2 *Interference or contraindication of other devices*

MRI can only be done under very restricted conditions.

Other surgeries: prophylactic antibiotic is recommended. Diathermy is strictly forbidden. Electrocoagulation should be restricted to bipolar mode.

Table 9.2 **Clinical outcomes of DBS**			
	STN	**GPi**	**Vim**
Off-motor symptoms	Improvement of 40–60%. *Decline over time (because progression of PD) but still effective after 5 years	Improvement of 26–56%. Decline of benefit after the first year	Improvement of tremor 70–90% maintained (5 years) Development of other symptoms over time
Dyskinesia	Improvement of 50%[†] Maintained over time	Improvement of 50–76%[‡] Maintained over time (4–5 years)	No effect
Dopaminergic medication	Reduction of 50%	No or little changes	No change

Machinery that can cause electromagnetic interference (security gates) should be avoided as they can turn off the stimulation. The new IPG generation are not likely to have this problem.

9.1.5 **Future of DBS: new targets**

There is a need to address symptoms that do not respond to stimulation of the current targets. Preliminary results of low frequency stimulation of the pedunculopontine nucleus for dopa-refractory gait and freezing have shown to be promising.

9.2 **Ablative procedures**

9.2.1 **Classical ablative procedures**

Ablative procedures consist on performing a permanent lesion within the selected target using thermocoagulation.

The interest in this procedure has declined since the introduction of DBS technology, since DBS provides less risk of side effects in particular for bilateral interventions. Bilateral lesions have mostly been abandoned and few centers carry out lesion procedures.

Unilateral lesions can be considered when:

• DBS technology is not available

• general anaesthesia is contraindicated

• the patient does not want implantable hardware and/or cannot suitably participate in the programming of the stimulation parameters; and

• hardware implantation is contraindicated (immunosuppresion).

Brain targets and patient selection criteria for ablative surgery are the same than those for DBS.

The operation is performed under local anaesthesia. Target coordinates and perioperative assessments are done in the same way as for DBS and a lesion is performed using different thermocoagulation protocols.

Unilateral pallidotomy and thalamotomy are the most frequently performed ablative procedures performed. Unilateral subthalamotomy is done only in few centers, some of them carrying out staged bilateral lesions.

The efficacy of unilateral procedures is similar to unilateral DBS for each target.

Side effects can not be adjustable as with DBS. The main side effects related to each target are:

• Pallidotomy: hemianopsia, dysarthria, dysphagia, gait difficulties and cognitive dysfunction

• Thalamotomy: ataxia, cognitive decline and dysarthria

- Subthalamotomy: postoperative chorea that usually resolves spontaneously during the first six months, although some patients may require pallidotomy to obtain complete control. Speech and balance are also at risk of deterioration.

9.2.2 Ablative procedures using radiosurgery (gamma knife)

Radiosurgery is a 'non-invasive' surgical option to create lesion in selected targets.

Currently the procedure is restricted to radiosurgical thalamotomy and it is done only in few centres.

It can be considered in patients where ablative or DBS procedures are contraindicated such as:

- elderly patients
- coagulopathies or anticoagulant treatment that cannot be discontinued
- other medical comorbidities
- extensive white matter changes or severe brain atrophy in the MRI.

9.3 Neuroprotective and neurorestorative surgical approaches

9.3.1 Cell transplantation

Transplantation of dopamine-producing cells has been explored during the last two decades in humans. Different approaches have been considered:

Striatal transplantation of autologous adrenal tissue. It was the first approach and was abandoned because the benefits were mild and transient, and it was associated with high mortality.

Striatal transplantation of fetal nigral cells. After positive results from preclinical and open label studies, two large randomized, placebo-controlled studies have been negative. Better results were found in a subgroup of patients (younger (age ≤ 60 years old), milder disease, and good response to levodopa at baseline). The main side effect is the occurrence of off-medication disabling dyskinesia.

Retinal pigment epithelial cells and carotid body glomus cells also produce dopamine and are currently under investigation.

Stem cells are pluripotent cells that can differentiate into dopamine neurons. So far stem cells research remains in a preclinical stage and several issues need to be resolved prior to clinical trials.

Recently it has been seen that grafted cells can also be affected by the disease pathology process, which might limit the long-term benefit of cell transplantation.

9.3.2 Trophic factors

Trophic factors are proteins that support and protect subpopulations of cells. Two main trophic factors have been investigated for PD in humans: Glial-derived neurotrophic factor (GDNF) and an analogue, neurturin. Both have been shown to have potential neuroprotective and neurorestorative actions in animal models of PD. Infusion of recombinant GDNF, showed benefits in a small open label study, that were not reproduced in a larger, randomized, placebo-controlled trial. Limited diffusion and immunological aspects seems to be its major disadvantages. New delivery systems might be explored in the future.

9.3.3 Gene therapy

Gene therapy involves insertion of a gene of interest into cells in order to change their function. The gene can be transferred into the appropriate brain region inserted in a viral vector (recombinant adeno-associated viral vector) or through transplantation of cells modified to express a therapeutic gene. Three gene therapy clinical trials are currently underway:

Neurturin, a trophic factor. After positive results in the phase I study, a phase II trial is in progress and results are expected in late 2008.

Glutamic acid decarboxylase (GAD). It is delivered into the STN. GAD catalyzes the biosynthesis of the inhibitory neurotransmitter γ-aminobutyric acid 'mimicking' the effect of DBS of this nucleus. A phase I study has been concluded with encouraging results.

Aromatic L-amino acid decarboxylase. It participates in the biosynthesis of dopamine. A phase I trial is ongoing.

9.4 Conclusion

There is at present no real surgical alternative to DBS. Advances in our understanding of molecular genetic and stem cells will help in the development of these therapies that might, in the future, replace DBS.

References and further reading

Deuschl G., Schade-Brittinger C., Krack P. *et al.* (2006) A Randomized Trial of Deep Brain Stimulation for Parkinson's disease. *N Engl J Med.* **355**, 896–908.

Freed C.R., Greene P.E., Breeze R.E. *et al.* (2001) Transplantation of embryonic dopamine neurons for severe Parkinson's disease. *N Engl J Med.* **344**, 710–19.

Gill S.S., Patel N.K., Hotton G.R. *et al.* (2003) Direct brain infusion of glial cell line-derived neurotrophic factor in Parkinson's disease. *Nat Med.* **9**, 589–95.

Kaplitt M.G., Feigin A., Tang C. et al. (2007) Safety and tolerability of gene therapy with an adeno-associated virus (AAV) borne GAD gene for Parkinson's disease: an open label, phase I trial. Lancet 369, 2097–2105.

Krack P., Fraix V, Mendes A., Benabid A.L., Pollak P. (2002) Postoperative management of subthalamic nucleus stimulation for Parkinson's Disease. Mov Disord. 17(3), S188–S197.

Krack P., Batir A., Van Blercom N. et al. (2003) Five-years follow-up of bilateral stimulation of the subthalamic nucleus in advanced Parkinson's disease. N Engl J Med. 349, 1925–34.

Laitinen L.V., Bergenheim A.T., Hariz M.I. (1992) Leksell's posteroventral pallidotomy in the treatment of Parkinson's disease. J Neurosurg. 76, 53–61.

Limousin P., Krack P., Pollak P., Benazzouz A., Ardouin C., Hoffmann D., Benabid A.L. (1998) Electrical stimulation of the subthalamic nucleus in advanced Parkinson's disease. N Engl J Med. 339, 1105–11.

Limousin P., Speelman J.D., Gielen F., Janssens M. (1999) Multicentre European study of thalamic stimulation in parkinsonian and essential tremor. J Neurol Neurosurg Psychiatry 66, 289–96.

Mazzone P., Lozano A., Stanzione P. et al. (2005) Implantation of human pedunculopontine nucleus: a safe and clinically relevant target in Parkinson's disease. Neuroreport., 16, 1877–81.

Mochizuki H., Yasuda T., Mouradian M.M. (2008) Advances in gene therapy for movement disorders. Neurotherapeutics. 5(2), 260–9.

Piccini P., Brooks D.J., Björklund A. et al. (1999) Dopamine release from nigral transplants visualized in vivo in a Parkinson's patient. Nat Neurosci. 2, 1137–40.

Plaha P., Gill S.S. (2005) Bilateral deep brain stimulation of the pedunculopontine nucleus for Parkinson's disease. Neuroreport. 16, 1883–7.

Rodriguez-Oroz M.C., Obeso J.A., Lang A.E. et al. (2005) Bilateral deep brain stimulation in Parkinson's disease: a multicentre study with 4 years follow-up. Brain, 128, 2240–9.

Volkmann J., Sturm V., Weiss P. et al. (1998) Bilateral high-frequency stimulation of the internal globus pallidus in advanced Parkinson's disease. Ann Neurol. 44, 953–61.

Acknowledgement

This work was undertaken at University College London Hospitals and University College London (UCLH/UCL) with a proportion of funding from the Department of Health's National Institute for Health Research (NIHR) Biomedical Research Centres funding scheme. The Unit of Functional Neurosurgery is supported by the Parkinson's Appeal. I.M.T. is supported by a Postgraduated Grant of the Fundacion Caja Madrid.

Chapter 10

Neuroprotection and disease-modification in Parkinson's disease

Olivier Rascol

Key points

- 'Neuroprotective' compounds blocking neuronal death mechanisms are expected to slow the progression of Parkinson's disease (PD) symptoms and to reduce patients' cumulative disability. This clinical effect is called 'disease-modification'.
- No drug has yet been approved for a 'disease-modification' indication in PD due to controversial trial designs (study duration, placebo comparison, clinical relevancy of endpoints, and confounding effect of symptomatic medications...) and negative or ambiguous results with various compounds including dopamine agonists, MAO-B inhibitors, and others
- In a recent 'delayed-start' trial (ADAGIO), rasagiline 1 mg daily early therapy provided a benefit on UPDRS scores that could not be equalled when the drug was introduced late. This is compatible with a 'disease-modification' effect but can be explained by other mechanisms than neuroprotection (enhanced compensation for example) and supports the concept of early management of PD patients with this drug
- Longer follow-up and pragmatic trials must be conducted to assess if the early but modest benefits detected in 'delayed-start' trials are clinically relevant on longer follow-up.

10.1 Summary

'Neuroprotective' compounds blocking dopamine neuronal death mechanisms are expected to slow the progression of Parkinson's disease (PD) symptoms and to reduce patients' cumulative disability. This objective is known as 'disease-modification'.

No drug has yet been approved for a 'disease-modification' indication. There are several reasons for this. Our understanding of neuron death remains partial, animal models are poorly predictive and neuroprotective candidates may target inadequate mechanisms. Moreover, attempts to demonstrate 'disease-modification' clinically is difficult because of the slow progression of PD and the shortcomings of study designs, including limited duration of patients' exposure to placebo, confounding effects of symptomatic antiparkinsonian medications and lack of reliable surrogate biomarkers.

Negative or at best ambiguous results have been obtained with most tested compounds including dopamine agonists and MAO-B inhibitors. However, a recent delayed-start trial (ADAGIO) showed that rasagiline 1 mg daily early therapy provides benefits that cannot be equalled with later therapy. This is compatible with 'disease-modification' effects (regardless of neuroprotective or enhanced compensatory mechanisms) and supports early management of PD patients with this drug. Pragmatic trials must be conducted to confirm that these early but modest benefits are clinically relevant on longer follow-up.

The term 'neuroprotection' refers to the enhancement of neuronal survival by blockade of cell death mechanisms. Many 'neuroprotective' agents enhancing in vitro or in vivo the survival of dopaminergic neurons have been identified under experimental conditions. Such compounds are expected, when given to patients with PD, to prevent them progressing to more advanced disease stages during which symptoms are more disabling. The term 'disease-modification' refers to this ambitious therapeutic objective, and to the capacity of a drug to slow the clinical progression of PD and reduce its cumulative disability. Within the last two decades, several 'neuroprotective' drugs have been assessed clinically to qualify as 'disease-modifiers', with at best mitigating results.

10.2 **Neuroprotective candidates for PD**

Our understanding of the cause(s) of PD has improved recently but the etiology of PD remains unknown. It probably involves the conjunction of environmental and genetic factors, leading to a cascade of pathophysiological events inducing dopaminergic neurons death. Factors identified as playing a role in this fatal cascade include increased levels of iron and monoamine oxidase (MAO)-B activity, glutamatergic excitotoxicity, nitric oxide synthesis, oxidative stress and depletion of antioxidants, inflammatory processes, abnormal protein folding and aggregation, reduced expression of trophic factors, altered calcium homeostasis, and apoptosis (Schapira et al. 2004).

Blockers of these deleterious mechanisms improve dopaminergic neurons survival in models of PD, including 1-methyl-4-phenyl-1, 2, 3, 6-tetrahydropyridine (MPTP) and 6-hydroxydopamine (6-OHDA). Neuroprotection can therefore be afforded with molecules like iron chelators, free radical scavenger antioxidants, MAO-B inhibitors, glutamate antagonists, nitric oxide synthetase inhibitors, calcium channel blockers, trophic factors, anti-apoptotic agents, etc, providing a large list of candidates for 'disease-modification' (Table 10.1).

10.3 'Disease-modification' trials in PD: methodological issues

Neuroprotection is a mechanistic concept. Counting neurons is not possible in vivo in humans and neurons might survive without functioning. Therefore, 'disease-modification' trials aim at demonstrating clinically relevant improvements in progression of cumulative disability (Sampaio and Rascol 2007). Designing such trials in PD is challenging, because the disorder progresses slowly and patients receive efficacious symptomatic medications 'masking' their symptoms.

A first difficulty is to rapidly evaluate the potential of a candidate, to avoid advancing ineffective (or inappropriately dosed) agents into large, long-term and expensive Phase III trials. For this purpose, Phase II 'proof-of-concept' 'futility' or 'adaptive' trial designs are proposed. The single-arm Phase II futility design uses a short-term outcome to

Table 10.1 Examples of 'neuroprotective' agents (with the main presumed neuroprotective mechanism(s) of action) that have been tested or are currently tested in Parkinson's disease as 'disease-modifier' candidates in 'disease-modification' trials (alphabetical order)

- CEP-1347 (antiapoptotic)
- CoEnzyme Q10 (improvement of mitochondrial function, indirect antioxidant)
- Creatine (improvement of mitochondrial function, indirect antioxidant)
- Dopamine agonists (bromocriptine, pramipexole, ropinirole) (antioxidants, antiapoptotic)
- GM1 ganglioside (potentiation of trophic factors, antiapoptotic)
- GPI 1485 (neuroimmunophilin) (mechanism uncertain)
- MAO-B inhibitors (rasagiline, selegiline) (blockers of MAO-B, antiapoptotic)
- Minocycline (antiinflammatory and antiapoptotic)
- Riluzole (antiglutamate)
- TCH346 (antiapoptotic)
- Tocopherol(Vitamine E) (antioxidant)
- Xaliproden (potentiation of trophic factor)

compare a treatment group response to a predetermined hypothesized, or historically based, control response and allows the identification of drugs that do not achieve the predefined success criteria (Tilley et al. 2006). The adaptive trial design allows trial design modifications to be made after patients have been enrolled, in order to increase trial flexibility without compromising its scientific method – for example, dropping a treatment arm, modifying the sample size, narrowing the trial focus, balancing treatment assignments using adaptive randomization, or stopping a study early due to success or failure (Müller and Schäfer 2001).

In Phase III, 'disease-modification' efficacy studies use a prospective, randomized, parallel-group, placebo-controlled, design, but controversial issues remain, including optimal target population, best choice for outcome measures, trial duration and disentanglement of 'symptomatic' from 'disease-modifying' effects.

10.3.1 **Target population**

Patients with PD progress from a pre-symptomatic/pre-motor ('at risk') stage to early untreated (de novo) symptomatic stage, stable treated 'symptomatic motor' stage, advanced stage with dopaminergic motor complications (fluctuations and dyskinesias) and late non-dopaminergic signs (autonomic dysfunction, falls, dementia, etc). Each stage offers advantages/disadvantages for 'disease-modification' assessment (Table 10.2), but the most commonly tested population is the early untreated symptomatic one. At this stage, 40–50% of dopaminergic neurons might be still alive and available for neuroprotective interventions. PD progression might be relatively rapid, allowing faster detection of modifying effects. A further advantage is that the measurement of disability is not confounded by the effects of previous/current symptomatic medications. This population, however, has disadvantages. Patients' disability may require rapid symptomatic therapy, making the treatment-free window between diagnosis and symptomatic therapy too narrow to detect a disease-modification effect. Maintaining patients on placebo may be unethical, generate high dropout rate and select slowly progressing patients. Another limitation is the limited recruitment of early patients, as PD incidence is low. The risk of misdiagnosis is not trivial at this stage, although diagnostic criteria are accepted as eligible by the regulatory agencies (EMEA, FDA). Another problem is that symptoms are modest in this early stage, while current clinical assessment scales are not optimally sensitive and the clinical relevance of mild disability changes is questionable. In addition, it is unknown whether a small change at this stage is predictive of long-term outcome.

Table 10.2 Advantages and disadvantages of the different stages of Parkinson's disease as target populations for a disease-modification trial

	Parkinson's disease stages			
	Pre-motor	Early un-treated	Stable treated	Advanced
Remaining neurons to protect	Many	Some	Few	Negligible
Progression of symptoms	Fast	Fast	Moderate	Slow
Recruitment of patients	?	Difficult	Easy	Easy
Diagnosis reliability	?	Poor	Moderate	Moderate
Use of symptomat-ic therapies	No	No	Yes	Yes
Motor fluctuations	No	No	(No)	Yes
Level of disability	None	Modest	Moderate	High

10.3.2 Outcome measures

As already stated, from a pragmatic perspective, a 'disease-modifier' should reduce clinical progression rate or, in other words, prevent or postpone disability in a clinically relevant and persistent manner.

Two main clinical endpoints are used to monitor PD disability over time in 'disease-modification' trials. The first one compares the rate of decline of progression of cardinal clinical features using the Unified Parkinson's Disease Rating Scale (UPDRS) (Fahn and Elton 1987). It is based on a slopes analysis approach to assess therapeutic efficacy. UPDRS (and its coming new version, MDS-UPDRS) is the best validated scale for PD (Goetz et al. 2007). In early untreated PD, its established annual rate of change is linear and equals 8–10 units. It is influenced by the use of symptomatic drugs and, once symptomatic treatment has been received, cannot be relied upon for the unbiased assessment of disease modification.

The time to emergence of clinically relevant milestones is another option. Survival curve models allow analyzing a treatment effect on such binary outcomes. The need for symptomatic dopaminergic therapy represents a level of disability that can be considered as clinically relevant and has been employed in several studies (Parkinson Study Group 1989). It can only be used in early untreated patients. In addition, there is the issue of which symptomatic treatment should be used as the marker (levodopa, dopamine agonists, MAO-B inhibitors, amantadine or anticholinergics), particularly as the delay to use these drugs is not standard and varies from investigator to investigator, some advocating delaying and others promoting early therapy based on various scientific, socio-cultural or economic factors (Schapira and Obeso 2006). The shift to Hoehn and Yahr stage III (emergence of balance problems) might be a more objective milestone, although an operational standardized definition is lacking (Hoehn and Yahr 1967). 'Balance problems' could be interpreted as anything from the first patient fall, to a variety of abnormalities observed in the pull test. This milestone has the advantage of being suitable for patients already on symptomatic medications because falls are generally considered as poorly responsive to dopaminergic therapies, although axial parkinsonian symptoms partly respond to levodopa. Moreover, balance problems may require years before occuring.

Functional imaging markers have also been explored to monitor PD progression, including the transformation of levodopa to dopamine using PET (18F-dopa) and the labeling of the dopamine transporter using SPECT (β-CIT) (Ravina *et al.* 2001). These biomarkers have some advantages over clinical endpoints: they are more objective, more sensitive, and presumably unaffected by symptomatic effects. However, they are expensive and do not explore non-dopamine degenerative processes. Inter-centre standardization is complex. Method validation issues remain, including the possible differential down-regulation of such biomarkers by levodopa versus other dopaminergic drugs. Finally, a major problem is that clinical validation (qualification) is not established as there are multiple examples of discrepancies between clinical outcome and neuroimaging changes. For example, embryonic mesencephalic cell implantation showed improved 18F-dopa PET signal without clinical benefit (Freed *et al.* 2001). This prevents using these biomarkers as surrogates endpoints in 'disease-modification' trials, although they can assist with early proof-of-concept and dose-finding trials, or provide support to understand mechanisms of action in Phase III.

10.3.3 **Duration of 'disease-modification' trials in PD**

A major methodological issue in PD 'disease-modification' trial design refers to study duration. Two temporal issues must be considered: (1) the optimal duration of the trial as PD progresses slowly, and (2) the disentanglement a 'short' symptomatic therapeutic response from a 'long-lasting' disease-modification effect.

10.3.3.1 *Disease-modification trials length*

The duration of a disease-modification trial depends on the expected treatment effect (greater effect, faster detection), the number of patients (more patients, greater power to detect small changes early) and the outcome measure (more precise, easier to detect small changes early). Increasing the number of patients allows a reduction in the duration of follow-up, but greater numbers of patients pose recruitment problems. One to two year follow-up of few hundred patients per treatment arm represents a common and feasible compromise. Placebo is the only possible comparator, but the maximal period that is feasible for placebo exposure in early patients (~9–12 months) is short to observe a disease-modification effect. Within this timeframe, disability changes are small and their clinical relevance questionable. Options to overcome these limitations include conducting pragmatic trials: the investigational disease-modifier is given as an add-on to stable symptomatic therapies in a large (thousands of patients) parallel-group, placebo-controlled trial lasting three to five years, and using simple global patient-rated endpoints (such as quality of life scales) that fit with routine clinical practice (Wheatley et al. 2002).

10.3.3.2 *Overcoming confounding symptomatic effects: short-term versus long-term effects*

A drug can delay disability outcomes in PD in two different ways – by preserving neuron health or by providing symptomatic control (or both). The duration of the observed effect help to separate these mechanisms, as 'short-lasting' improvement indicates a symptomatic effect, while a 'long-lasting' response indicates a neuroprotective effect. Two main study designs have been proposed in an attempt to disentangle these mechanisms and eliminate the impact of symptomatic effects:

Wash-out design: this design aims to eliminate confounding symptomatic effects by including a period of medication withdrawal after a period of active treatment (Parkinson Study Group 1993), (Fahn et al. 2004). If a benefit is seen in the active arm at the end of the follow-up period and persists after the wash-out period, this indicates a long-lasting disease-modification response (Figure 10.1). The problem here is the duration of the wash-out. For example, levodopa has a 90-minute elimination half-life, while its clinical antiparkinsonian response can last for several weeks after withdrawal. A wash-out period of more than a few days is unethical and causes high drop-out numbers. Too short wash-out duration is insufficient to eliminate a confounding long-duration symptomatic effect, leading to inconclusive interpretations.

Delayed-start design: in this design, patients are randomized to initiate treatment with study drug (early-start) or placebo for a fixed time interval (Phase A). The placebo group is then switched to active treatment (delayed-start), and both groups are followed for another fixed time interval to let the symptomatic effect equilibrate into the two arms, regardless of the start time (Phase B) (Olanow et al. 2008). Differences between the two groups at the end of Phase A can be due to symptomatic and/or neuroprotective effects. However, if the difference observed at the end of Phase A disappears at

Figure 10.1 The wash-out study design and its possible outcomes

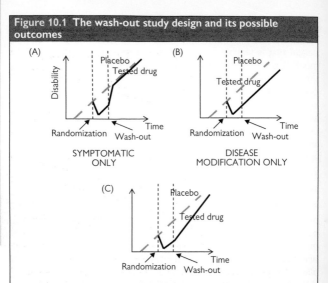

In all three panels, the tested medication improves disability as compared with placebo. However, once washed-out, patient outcomes vary according to the different scenarios.

A. SYMPTOMATIC ONLY: disability improvement in the active group is short-lasting and disappears after drug withdrawal. This is in suggestive of a symptomatic response with no disease-modification effect.

B. DISEASE-MODIFICATION ONLY: disability improvement persists in the active group, even after drug withdrawal. This is in favour of a long-lasting 'disease-modification effect'.

C. INCONCLUSIVE: curves tend to join after wash-out, but do not catch-up during the trial follow-up. This can be interpreted either as a long-lasting symptomatic effect requiring longer wash-out, or a mixed symptomatic and disease-modification effect.

the end of Phase B, this indicates a solely symptomatic effect (Figure 10.2). Conversely, if the difference is sustained and the delayed-start group does not catch up with the early-start group, this means that early treatment conferred a benefit that cannot simply be explained by a symptomatic effect. Delayed-start trials are powered to detect small UPDRS differences because of limited placebo phase duration. These small changes may not be clinically significant or sustained, and require further longer studies to assess whether any difference is maintained. Finally, a positive result in the early treatment group might not necessarily mean that the drug exerted a 'neuroprotective' effect, but may have simply helped maintaining basal ganglia compensatory mechanisms or preventing maladaptive responses.

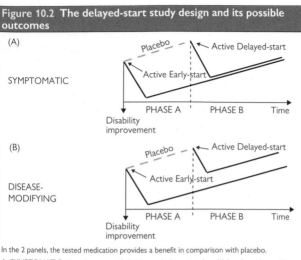

Figure 10.2 The delayed-start study design and its possible outcomes

(A)

SYMPTOMATIC

Placebo

Active Delayed-start

Active Early-start

PHASE A | PHASE B | Time

Disability improvement

(B)

DISEASE-MODIFYING

Placebo

Active Delayed-start

Active Early-start

PHASE A | PHASE B | Time

Disability improvement

In the 2 panels, the tested medication provides a benefit in comparison with placebo.

A. SYMPTOMATIC: the substitution of placebo with the active drug (delayed-start) provides a benefit that allows the group to 'catch-up' with the early-start group, with similar improvement at the end of Phase B. This is in favour of a purely symptomatic effect.

B. DISEASE-MODIFYING: the delayed introduction of tested drug after placebo does not provide a benefit equal to that observed when patients start active treatment early, and the difference persists throughout Phase B. Patients starting treatment early did better than those who started late, and this cannot be explained by a pure symptomatic effect. This is in favour of a 'disease-modification' effect, regardless of underlying mechanisms ('neuroprotection' or enhancement of early compensatory mechanisms). An alternative reflection of such a disease modifying effect is the reduced slope of progression (i.e. slower) of motor deficit in the early start group.

10.4 Examples of 'disease-modification' trials in PD

It is beyond the scope of this chapter to extensively review all different 'disease-modification' trials conducted in PD. Overall, in 2008, none have provided sufficient evidence to conclude that any drug offers a clinically-relevant and long-lasting 'disease-modification' effect. However, some encouraging, although questionable results have been obtained.

Riluzole (Olanow *et al.* 2002), TCH346 (Olanow *et al.* 2006), CEP-1347 (Parkinson Study Group 2007) or Vitamin E7, for example, clearly failed to delay time to dopaminergic therapy in placebo-controlled parallel randomized studies conducted in untreated patients with early PD, thus excluding any potential disease-modifying effect at the tested doses.

Positive signals, compatible with a disease-modification effect, have been obtained with drugs like selegiline, Coenzyme Q10, levodopa, pramipexole or ropinirole. These trials remain however inconclusive because of intrinsic ambiguous interpretations. Selegiline significantly delayed the need for levodopa versus placebo in early untreated PD patients in the DATATOP trial (Parkinson Study Group 1993). This effect can however be at least partly explained by the symptomatic effect of the drug, preventing firm establishment of any 'disease-modification' response in this case. Untreated early PD patients receiving levodopa for 40 weeks had better UPDRS scores than those randomized to placebo after 15 days of wash-out at the end of the ELLDOPA trial (Fahn *et al.* 2004). Unfortunately, this short wash-out period might have not been long enough to clear-out all symptomatic benefit of levodopa. So it was not possible to conclude that levodopa modified PD progression. After two to four-year follow-up, neuroimaging dopaminergic biomarkers (18F-DOPA and beta-CIT) declined less in early de novo PD patients on dopamine agonists (pramipexole or ropinirole) than levodopa (Parkinson Study Group 2002), (Whone *et al.*). This finding may be interpreted as indicative of a 'neuroprotective' effect of the agonists, but it is also possible that levodopa down-regulated these biomarkers more profoundly than the agonists, preventing any firm interpretation. More recently, two delayed-start 'disease-modification' trials (TEMPO, ADAGIO) showed consistently that patients starting early on rasagiline did better on UPDRS scores than those starting six to nine months later (Parkinson Study Group 2004; Rascol and Olanow 2008). This is encouraging, in favour of a possible 'disease-modifying' effect of rasagiline, but it remains uncertain if the difference observed at the end of this 18-month trial (less than 2 points in total UPDRS score) is clinically relevant and will persist after longer follow-up (Clarke 2008).

10.5 **Conclusions**

In summary, no medication has yet demonstrated relevant 'disease-modification' properties based on undisputable clinical evidence (Movement Disorder Society task force 2002; Goetz *et al.* 2005). A better understanding of dopaminergic cell death mechanisms and more accurate experimental models of PD accounting for pathophysiological factors other than the sole dopaminergic ones (brain compensatory plasticity and non-dopaminergic neuronal loss) should help identify better neuroprotective candidates for 'disease-modification' strategies. In parallel, better designed clinical trials should help in assessing these 'disease-modification' effects. Presently, regardless of our understanding of the possible underlying mechanisms of action, we need drugs that provide robust and sustained reduction in patients' cumulative disability. Once identified, such 'disease-modifiers' should certainly be used as early as possible to manage our patients.

References and further reading

Clarke C.E. (2008) Are delayed-start design trials to show neuroprotection in Parkinson's disease fundamentally flawed? *Mov Disord.* **23**(6), 784–9.

Fahn S., Elton R., members of the UPDRS Development Committee. (1987) Unified Parkinson's Disease Rating Scale. In: Fahn S., Marsden C.D., Calne D.B., Goldstein M. (eds). Recent Developments in Parkinson's Disease. Volume II. Macmillan Health Care Information, Florham Park, NJ, USA.

Fahn S., Oakes D., Shoulson I., *et al.* (2004) Parkinson Study Group. Levodopa and the progression of Parkinson's disease. *N Engl J Med.* **351**(24), 2498–2508.

Freed C.R., Greene P.E., Breeze R.E., *et al.* (2001) Transplantation of embryonic dopamine neurons for severe Parkinson's disease. *N Engl J Med.* **344**(10), 710–19.

Goetz C.G., Fahn S., Martinez-Martin P., *et al.* (2007) Movement Disorder Society-sponsored revision of the Unified Parkinson's Disease Rating Scale (MDS-UPDRS): Process, format, and clinimetric testing plan. *Mov Disord.* **22**(1), 41–7.

Goetz C.G., Poewe W., Rascol O., Sampaio C. (2005) Evidence-based medical review update: pharmacological and surgical treatments of Parkinson's disease: 2001 to 2004. *Mov Disord.* **20**(5), 523–39.

Hoehn M.M., Yahr M.D. (1967) Parkinsonism: onset, progression and mortality. *Neurology* **17**(5), 427–42.

Movement Disorder Society task force (2002) Management of Parkinson's disease: an evidence-based review. *Mov Disord.* **17**(4), S1–S166.

Müller H.H., Schäfer H. (2001) Adaptive group sequential designs for clinical trials: combining the advantages of adaptive and classical group sequential approaches. *Biometrics* **57**(3), 886–91.

Olanow C.W., Rascol O., Hauser R., *et al.* (2009) A double-blind, delayed-start trial of rasagline in Parkinson's disease. *N Engl J Med* **361**(13), 1268–78.

Olanow C.W., Schapira A.H., LeWitt P.A., Kieburtz K., Sauer D., Olivieri G., Pohlmann H., Hubble J. (2006) TCH346 as a neuroprotective drug in Parkinson's disease: a double-blind, randomised, controlled trial. *Lancet Neurol.* **5**(12), 1013–20.

Parkinson Study Group PRECEPT Investigators. (2007) Mixed lineage kinase inhibitor CEP-1347 fails to delay disability in early Parkinson disease. *Neurology* **69**(15), 1480–90.

Parkinson Study Group. (1989) Effect of deprenyl on the progression of disability in early Parkinson's disease. *N Engl J Med.* **321**(20), 1364–71.

Parkinson Study Group (1993) Effects of tocopherol and deprenyl on the progression of disability in early Parkinson's disease. *N Engl J Med.* **328**(3), 176–83.

Parkinson Study Group. (2002) Dopamine transporter brain imaging to assess the effects of pramipexole vs levodopa on Parkinson disease progression. *JAMA* **287**(13), 1653–61.

Parkinson Study Group (2004) A controlled, randomized, delayed-start study of rasagiline in early Parkinson disease. *Arch Neurol.*, **61**(4), 561–6.

Rascol O., Olanow C.W., Brooks D., *et al.* (2002) A 2-year multicenter placebo-controlled, double-blind parallel group study of the effect of riluzole in Parkinson's disease. *Mov Disord.* **17**, 39.

Rascol O., Olanow W.C. (2008) ADAGIO: A prospective, double-blind, delayed-start study to examine the disease-modifying effect of rasagiline in early Parkinsons disease (PD). *Eur J Neurol.* **15**(3), 413.

Ravina B., Eidelberg D., Ahlskog J.E., *et al.* (2001) The role of radiotracer imaging in Parkinson disease. *Neurology* **64**(2), 208–15.

Sampaio C., Rascol O. (2007) Disease-modification strategies in Parkinson's disease. In: Jankovic J., Tolosa E. (eds) *Parkinson's Disease and Movement Disorders.* 5th edn. Lippincott Williams & Wilkins, Philadelphia, USA.

Schapira A.H., Olanow C.W. (2004) Neuroprotection in parkisnon's disease: mysteries, myths, and misconceptions. *JAMA* **2914**(3), 358–64.

Schapira A.H., Obeso J. (2006) Timing of treatment initiation in Parkinson's disease: a need for reappraisal? *Ann Neurol.* **259**(3), 559–62.

Tilley B.C., Palesch Y.Y., Kieburtz K., *et al.* (2006) NET-PD Investigators. Optimizing the ongoing search for new treatments for Parkinson disease: using futility designs. *Neurology* **266**(5), 628–33.

Wheatley K., Stowe R.L., Clarke C.E., Hills R.K., Williams A.C., Gray R. (2002) Evaluating drug treatment for Parkinson's disease: how good are the trials? *BMJ* **324**(7352), 1508–11.

Whone A.L., Watts R.L., Stoessl A.J., *et al.* (2003) REAL-PET Study Group. Slower progression of Parkinson's disease with ropinirole versus levodopa: the REAL-PET study. *Ann Neurol.* **54**(1), 93–101.

Index